Thrive with Osteoporosis

Your Guide to Prevent Fractures, Build Strength, Improve Balance, Embrace Natural Remedies, and Practice Safe Exercises for Lifelong Mobility

Isabella Harmony

Table of Contents

Introduction 9

Chapter 1: Understanding Osteoporosis.............................11

    Preventative Measures for Osteopenia:...........................12

    Understanding Osteoporosis...12

    Osteoporosis in Men vs. Women....................................13

    The Stages of Osteoporosis 14

Chapter 2: Diagnosis and Medical Testing..........................17

    Self-Assessment Tools 17

    Diagnostic Tools and Techniques...................................18

    Diagnosis and Medical Testing.......................................18

    Understanding Bone Density Scans (DEXA) 19

    Case Studies..19

    Jane - Rediscovering Strength Through Community Support............19

    Michael - A Firefighter's Path to Recovery and Prevention 20

    Maria - Traditional Wisdom Meets Modern Medicine.......................21

    Imani - Advocacy Through Adversity..............................22

    Ayesha - Bridging Cultures to Find Balance 23

    John - Late Diagnosis and the Path to Recovery 24

    Monitoring Bone Health..24

    Discussing Results with Your Doctor...............................26

Chapter 3: Medical Treatments and Alternatives...................29

    Overview of Osteoporosis Medications 30

    Types of Osteoporosis Medications 31

    Anabolic Therapies for Bone Building.............................32

    Natural Supplements: Calcium and Vitamin D 32

    Exploring Global Natural Remedies................................33

Chapter 4: Nutrition for Bone Health.................................35

Calcium-Rich Foods and How to Include them in your Diet..............37

Calcium-Rich Smoothie Bowl..38

Baked Salmon with Sesame Kale..39

Chickpea, Spinach, and Quinoa Stir-Fry......................................40

Tofu and Broccoli Stir-Fry with Almonds......................................41

Sardine and Avocado Toast 42

Almond Butter and Banana Chia Pudding....................................43

The Importance of Vitamin D 44

Spinach and Feta Stuffed Chicken Breast 45

Greek Yogurt Parfait with Almonds and Berries............................46

Roasted Brussels Sprouts with Tahini Drizzle 47

Calcium-Packed Veggie Pizza..48

Tofu Scramble with Kale and Mushrooms 49

Sweet Potato and Black Bean Tacos 50

Sardine Pasta with Lemon and Capers..51

Cottage Cheese and Berry Bowl...52

Broccoli and Cheddar Soup...53

Kale and White Bean Salad...54

Almond and Fig Overnight Oats 55

Spinach and Ricotta Stuffed Shells 56

Lentil and Sweet Potato Stew 57

Cabbage and Carrot Slaw with Tahini Dressing............................58

Baked Eggplant Parmesan..59

Sesame-Crusted Tofu Nuggets 60

Baked Oatmeal with Almonds and Berries 61

Swiss Chard and Mushroom Frittata 62

Orange and Almond Salad...63

Spaghetti Squash with Creamy Tahini Sauce...............................64

Creamy Polenta with Roasted Vegetables 65

Indian-Style Spinach and Paneer Curry (Saag Paneer)....................66

Mediterranean Chickpea and Tahini Salad 67

Japanese Miso Soup with Tofu and Wakame................................68

Mexican Black Bean and Avocado Tostadas 69

Greek Spanakopita (Spinach Pie) 70

West African Peanut Stew 71

Italian White Bean and Kale Bruschetta.......................................72

Korean Kimchi Fried Rice...73

Chapter 5: Exercise and Mobility 75

The Importance of Physical Activity...75

Weight-Bearing Exercises Explained 76

Balance and Coordination Training 77

Safe and Effective Strength Training 78

Safety Adaptations in Yoga and Pilates...80

Creating a Personalized Exercise Plan..80

Your Personal Movement Journey 81

Myth-Busting: Exercise and Osteoporosis 82

Practical Exercise Planning: A Step-by-Step Guide 82

Step 1: Professional Consultation...82

Step 2: Assessing Your Current Fitness Level 82

Step 3: Creating Your Personalized Exercise Toolkit.......................83

Step 4: Building Your Weekly Exercise Routine 83

Beginner's Weekly Template 83

Progression Strategies...84

Beginner Level (0-3 Months)..84

Intermediate Level (3-6 Months) 85

Advanced Level (6-12 Months) 85

Safety Red Flags: When to Stop 85

Technology and Exercise Support 85

Recommended Apps..85

Tracking Progress..86

Psychological Aspects of Exercise 86

Motivation Techniques 86

Mental Health Benefits..86

Your Movement, Your Power...86

Recommended Resources 86

Staying Motivated and Consistent...87

Chapter 6: Preventing Falls and Injuries.....................................89

Home Safety Modifications 89

Fall-Proofing Your Living Space..90

Assistive Devices and Technology 91

Safe Movement and Daily Activities 91

Emergency Preparedness for Falls...92

Importance of Routine Vision and Hearing Checks 92

Practicing Mindful Movement 92

Chapter 7: Emotional Well-being and Support 93

Reflection Section: Self-Compassion Practice 94

Building a Support Network 94

Interactive Element: Support Network Checklist 95

The Role of Mental Health in Physical Health............................96

Resource List: Mental Health Resources...................................96

Planning for Long-Term Health 96

Resource List: Ongoing Support 97

Celebrating Progress and Setting Future Goals 97

Interactive Element: Milestone Celebration Ideas 97

Chapter 8: Staying Informed and Engaged............................99

Interactive Element: Research Spotlight........................100

Advocacy and Raising Awareness 100

Exploring Cutting-Edge Treatments 101

Expanding Lifestyle Modifications Beyond Diet and Exercise..........102

The Role of Digital Health Tools....................................102

Interactive Element: Digital Tools and Telemedicine 103

Chapter 9: Osteoporosis and Coexisting Conditions.........................105

Osteoarthritis (OA) and Osteoporosis: Managing Joint and Bone Health Together 105

Rheumatoid Arthritis (RA) and Osteoporosis: Navigating Immune and Bone Health..106

Type 2 Diabetes and Osteoporosis: Balancing Blood Sugar and Bone Health 106

Celiac Disease and Osteoporosis: Supporting Bone Health Through Diet 107

Chronic Kidney Disease (CKD) and Osteoporosis: Balancing Bone Health and Kidney Function...108

Depression and Osteoporosis: Prioritizing Mental and Bone Health108

Conclusion..113

References 117

Introduction

When my mom was diagnosed with osteoporosis, it was like being thrown off balance, like the entire floor was pulled out from under us. She was a pillar in our family, always lively and energetic. The diagnosis was made after a minor fall, which resulted in a fracture of the bone. I saw her suffer from pain, physical disability, and the stress that comes with the disability. It was not only heartbreaking, but it also became a turning point for the whole family. Her story motivated me to learn more about osteoporosis and how I could help her and other sufferers improve their quality of life.

This book is a result of that experience. My goal is to give you all the information you need on how to live with and effectively manage osteoporosis. We will explore all aspects of it, including the medical aspect of the disease, practical tips, natural remedies, and expert advice. I want to present authentic clinical information, emotions, and personal experiences that can help improve the quality of life daily.

Osteoporosis is indeed a complicated condition, but the first step towards managing it is knowing as much as possible about it. This book will help you understand the condition, who is most likely to be affected, and how it can be diagnosed. We will review the most recent research on traditional treatments and natural remedies and present a fair view of your choices.

This book is intended for anyone who is an adult with a diagnosis of osteoporosis, people who may be at risk of developing it, and caregivers who support them. Osteoporosis is not gender selective; it occurs in both men and women. My focus is to provide the most comprehensive guide possible for anyone who has to deal with this condition.

My motivation for writing this book stems from my mom's journey, but it's also driven by extensive research. I have invested my time and numerous hours in reading up-to-date studies and collecting data from around the world. I want to help you, not confuse you with too many medical terminologies. The information is easy to understand, and the emphasis is placed on recommended strategies that can be applied in everyday life.

Now, let's discuss what you will find in the chapters ahead. First, we will examine osteoporosis, how it impacts your bones, and who will most likely develop it. The next section will discuss today's medical treatment, including medications and surgical options. We will also take a look at dietary recommendations and provide recipes that are healthy as well as tasty. Physical activity is critical in osteoporosis prevention; we will guide you through safe exercises at home. We will also discuss measures to avoid falls, emotional well-being, and ways to stay updated with the latest research.

Some recommendations that can be drawn from this book include how to handle osteoporosis, how to avoid fractures, and how to enhance bone health through nutrition and physical exercises. You will also read tips on seeking emotional support from family and friends or hiring a professional to help you. The aim is to equip you with adequate knowledge and tools to lead an active life despite osteoporosis.

To ensure that the information provided in this book is as accurate and up-to-date as possible, I've conducted extensive customer research and read the most recent scientific studies. I hope that it will be of use to you and that you will be able to refer to it anytime you feel the need for some assistance. Osteoporosis affects your lifestyle in many ways but does not dictate how you should live. If you have the knowledge and the right tools, you can take control of your bone health and continue to lead an active lifestyle. I assure you that you are not alone on this journey.

Chapter 1: Understanding Osteoporosis

A few years ago, I watched my mom struggle with everyday tasks after being diagnosed with osteoporosis. A simple fall broke her wrist, and from then on, our lives were filled with doctor visits, medications, and the constant worry of her falling again. That experience inspired me to learn all I could about osteoporosis. This book is built on her strength and our journey together, and I hope to guide you through yours.

Osteoporosis is a condition that weakens bones, making them fragile and prone to fractures from even minor trauma. Imagine bones as solid structures, like buildings. In osteoporosis, this structure deteriorates, losing density and strength. Healthy bones have a dense, honeycomb-like pattern, while osteoporotic bones have larger spaces within the honeycomb, making them weaker and more prone to break.

Osteoporosis affects millions worldwide, predominantly older adults. The International Osteoporosis Foundation estimates around 200 million people have the condition globally, with about 10 million in the U.S. alone. An additional 44 million Americans are at risk due to low bone density. Women, particularly postmenopausal women, are more affected, though men can develop it too, especially as they age. The economic and social costs are vast, with billions spent on healthcare and the significant impact of fractures leading to long-term disability and loss of independence.

A key challenge with osteoporosis is that it often has no symptoms until a fracture occurs. Common sites for fractures are the hip, spine, and wrist. Hip fractures usually require surgery and can lead to long-term disability, while vertebral fractures can cause chronic pain and height loss. Though wrist fractures are less severe, they still hinder daily tasks. Over time, osteoporosis can result in chronic pain, limited mobility, reliance on caregivers, and even increasing mortality rates.

It's important to differentiate between osteoporosis and osteopenia. Osteopenia is a less severe condition where bone density is below average but not as low as osteoporosis. Think of it as a warning sign that bones are weakening. Without intervention, osteopenia can progress into osteoporosis.

Preventative Measures for Osteopenia:

- Eat a balanced diet rich in calcium and vitamin D.

- Engage in regular weight-bearing exercise.

- Avoid smoking and excessive alcohol consumption.

Understanding Osteoporosis

Understanding osteoporosis is crucial for managing it effectively. By recognizing its impact on bones and knowing the signs to watch for, you can take proactive steps to protect your bone health. In the following sections, we'll explore treatments, diet, exercise plans, and strategies to prevent falls and fractures, helping you lead an active life despite osteoporosis.

Bones may seem rigid, but they constantly undergo remodeling. Made of collagen and calcium phosphate, bones gain flexibility from collagen and strength from calcium phosphate. Think of collagen as steel bars and calcium phosphate as concrete, forming a sturdy structure that supports the body.

Bone remodeling involves two key cell types: osteoclasts (which break down old bone) and osteoblasts (which build new bone). The balance between these processes maintains bone density. When disrupted, bone density decreases, leading to osteoporosis.

Bone density refers to the amount of minerals in bone tissue. The higher the density, the stronger the bones. Bone density is typically measured using a DEXA scan, which compares your bone density to that of a young, healthy person. A low score indicates osteopenia or osteoporosis, helping guide treatment decisions.

Several factors influence bone density, including family history, hormonal changes, and nutrition. Estrogen protects bones, so bone loss accelerates after menopause. A diet rich in calcium and vitamin D and regular weight-bearing exercise promotes healthy bones. Smoking and excessive alcohol consumption harm bone health, and conditions like rheumatoid arthritis and diabetes can also lead to bone loss over time.

Osteoporosis develops gradually and is influenced by both uncontrollable and controllable risk factors. Age and gender are primary risks—women, especially postmenopausal women, are at higher risk due to hormonal changes. Men also experience bone density loss but at a slower rate. Family history plays a role, and hormonal imbalances can weaken bones.

Lifestyle factors like poor nutrition, lack of physical activity, smoking, and excessive alcohol consumption also increase osteoporosis risk. A diet low in calcium and vitamin D deprives bones of essential nutrients, while weight-bearing exercises help maintain bone strength. Diseases like rheumatoid arthritis and diabetes, along with medications such as corticosteroids, can negatively affect bone health.

To reduce risk, focus on proper nutrition, including calcium-rich foods like leafy greens and dairy, and ensure adequate vitamin D through sunlight, food, or supplements. Regularly engage in weight-bearing exercise and strength training. Quitting smoking and limiting alcohol can also improve bone health.

Regular screening for osteoporosis is recommended, especially for those over 50 or with risk factors. Early detection through bone density tests can guide prevention and treatment strategies to minimize fractures and bone loss.

Taking steps to address these risk factors, making lifestyle changes, and working closely with healthcare providers are crucial to maintaining bone health and preventing osteoporosis.

Osteoporosis in Men vs. Women

Osteoporosis affects both sexes but is more common in postmenopausal women due to hormonal changes. Estrogen plays a crucial role in maintaining bone density by inhibiting osteoclasts, the cells responsible for bone breakdown. As estrogen levels drop during menopause, bone loss accelerates. In men, testosterone supports bone health by promoting osteoblast function, the cells that build new bone. While men's testosterone levels decline with age (andropause), this process is slower than women's postmenopausal bone loss.

Fracture patterns also differ between genders. Women commonly experience fractures in the spine, hip, and wrist, while men are more likely to suffer from hip and spine fractures. Women lose bone density rapidly in the early postmenopausal years, whereas men experience a gradual decline.

Hormone Replacement Therapy (HRT) is often recommended for women to slow bone loss post-menopause, though it comes with risks and requires a doctor's supervision. Men may be prescribed testosterone replacement therapy if needed, but this also requires careful monitoring due to potential side effects.

Acknowledging these gender-specific differences is essential for developing effective treatment and prevention strategies, ensuring that men and women receive the care they need to maintain strong bones and an active lifestyle.

The Stages of Osteoporosis

Osteoporosis progresses in stages, with each phase presenting different signs and symptoms. Early recognition and treatment are key to managing the disease effectively.

1. **Osteopenia:** The first stage, characterized by mildly reduced bone density, is often symptomless and detected through bone density tests. Osteopenia signals the need for preventative measures, like increasing calcium and vitamin D intake and regular weight-bearing exercises, to slow further bone loss.
2. **Early Osteoporosis:** In this stage, bone density has declined further, but symptoms may still be absent. Many people discover they have osteoporosis after a minor fracture. Early intervention through medication and lifestyle changes can prevent progression.
3. **Advanced Osteoporosis:** In the final stage, bones are fragile and prone to fractures from minor stress, like bending or coughing. Symptoms include chronic pain, height loss, and kyphosis (hunched back), which significantly affect mobility and quality of life. Multifaceted treatment—including medications, physical therapy, and pain management—becomes essential.

Diagnosis involves measuring bone density using a DEXA scan. A T-score between -1.0 and -2.5 indicates osteopenia, while a score below -2.5 points to osteoporosis. Severe osteoporosis is diagnosed when this low score is paired with a history of fractures.

Treatment depends on the stage of the disease. In osteopenia, lifestyle modifications can prevent further bone loss. Early osteoporosis is managed with medications like bisphosphonates or SERMs to preserve bone density and reduce fracture risk. In advanced stages, treatment focuses on medications, physical therapy, fall prevention, and in some cases, surgery to repair fractures.

Understanding these stages and their associated symptoms allows for better management of osteoporosis and helps in implementing timely interventions to maintain bone health and quality of life.

Living with osteoporosis can be emotionally challenging. The constant fear of falling and breaking a bone creates persistent anxiety, which can lead to chronic stress, further worsening the condition. Many patients feel overwhelmed by their diagnosis, experiencing a loss of control that can contribute to depression.

Osteoporosis also affects social interactions. Activities once enjoyed, like dancing or hiking, may now feel too risky, leading to social withdrawal and isolation. This avoidance of social activities can strain relationships with family and friends, and relying on others for support can sometimes lead to feelings of being a burden.

Managing these emotional challenges is essential. Stress relief techniques, such as deep breathing, mindfulness, and progressive muscle relaxation, can help reduce anxiety. Building a strong support network of family, friends, or members of a local support group can provide both emotional and practical help. Seeking professional counseling, particularly Cognitive Behavioral Therapy (CBT), can be especially effective in managing anxiety and depression linked to chronic illness.

Chapter 2: Diagnosis and Medical Testing

Imagine waking up with a sharp pain in your back, dismissing it as part

of aging or an awkward night's sleep. Weeks pass, and the pain persists. You notice your jeans don't fit like they used to, despite no weight gain. You've lost height. These subtle changes are how osteoporosis often begins—quietly and without fanfare.

Osteoporosis is often called the "silent disease" because early stages typically have no symptoms. One of the first signs is unexplained, persistent back pain, which may result from undetected micro-fractures in the spine. Over time, this can lead to a hunched posture and severe back issues.

Another early indicator is gradual height loss, caused by the weakening and compression of spinal vertebrae. You may notice that reaching for high shelves becomes more complicated or that your clothes seem longer. Additionally, fractures from low-impact activities—like slipping on a rug or bending over—are warning signs that your bones are becoming less dense.

Women, especially postmenopausal, are more prone to these symptoms due to hormonal changes, while men experience a slower decline in bone density. Men may not realize they have osteoporosis until a fracture occurs, often later in life, leading to delayed diagnosis and treatment. Detecting these signs early allows for timely intervention, helping preserve bone strength and prevent fractures.

Self-Assessment Tools

Self-assessment tools, including online risk calculators, can help you gauge your osteoporosis risk by asking about factors like age, gender, family history, and past fractures. While these tools can't replace professional advice, they can prompt a discussion with your doctor. Additionally, checklists can guide you in discussing symptoms with your healthcare provider, ensuring you address all critical aspects such as diet, physical activity, and recent physical changes.

Early diagnosis and proactive treatment can make a significant difference in managing osteoporosis, preventing further bone deterioration, and supporting a healthier, more active life.

Diagnostic Tools and Techniques

The most commonly used diagnostic tool for osteoporosis is the DEXA scan, which measures bone mineral density (BMD). It provides clear images of areas most prone to fractures, such as the spine, hip, and forearm, allowing doctors to assess bone health and determine the necessary treatment plan.

Another diagnostic tool is quantitative ultrasound, which uses sound waves to assess bone density, typically on the heel. It's more affordable and portable than the DEXA scan, making it convenient for preliminary assessments. However, it's not as accurate as DEXA, and if results indicate low bone density, your doctor will likely recommend a DEXA scan for a more precise evaluation.

CT scans (computed tomography) can also measure bone density but are less commonly used due to higher radiation exposure and cost. These scans provide detailed images of bone structure and density. They are typically reserved for cases where other tests are inconclusive or when more precise imaging is needed, such as for surgical planning.

Peripheral bone density tests assess bone density in peripheral areas of the body, such as the wrist, fingers, or heel. These tests are faster and cheaper than the central DEXA scans but are less detailed. They can be used for preliminary assessments or in cases where a full-body DEXA scan is not possible. However, they should not be used as the only method to determine the presence of osteoporosis.

Magnetic resonance imaging, commonly known as MRI, can give you images of bones without having to use radiation. Although MRI is not widely used to diagnose osteoporosis, it can help determine the quality of the bone and identify fractures that cannot be seen on X-rays or DEXA scans. It helps give a detailed view of the structure of bones, which can be quite beneficial in formulating treatment plans.

Diagnosis and Medical Testing

The DEXA scan is the gold standard for diagnosing osteoporosis due to its accuracy in evaluating bone mineral density (BMD) at critical sites like the spine and hip. While it involves low radiation levels, it offers the most precise assessment of bone health. In contrast, quantitative ultrasound is a quicker, more affordable option without radiation but is less accurate and primarily used for initial screening. CT scans and MRIs provide detailed bone images but come with higher costs and radiation exposure.

The type of diagnostic tool used depends on individual risk factors. A DEXA scan is usually recommended for its precision in high-risk individuals. Ultrasound and peripheral bone density tests may serve as screening tools, especially when DEXA scans are unavailable. CT scans or MRIs may be used in more complex cases requiring detailed imaging.

Understanding Bone Density Scans (DEXA)

A DEXA scan uses two X-ray beams to measure bone density. It focuses on areas prone to fractures, such as the hips and spine, and is a noninvasive, pain-free procedure. Results include T-scores and Z-scores, which help assess the risk of fractures and guide treatment. While there are concerns about radiation, the exposure from a DEXA scan is minimal—lower than that from a chest X-ray.

The T-score compares your bone density to that of a young, healthy individual, while the Z-score compares it to others of your age, sex, and height. A T-score of -1.0 or higher is normal, while a lower score indicates bone loss. Bone turnover markers, such as alkaline phosphatase and osteocalcin, can provide additional insights into bone metabolism, helping assess treatment effectiveness.

Case Studies

Jane - Rediscovering Strength Through Community Support

At 52, Jane was diagnosed with osteoporosis after experiencing a wrist fracture from a minor fall. The news was shocking; she had always led an active lifestyle and assumed her bones were strong. Jane's first reaction was fear—fear of more fractures, fear of losing her independence, and fear of what the diagnosis meant for her future. However, Jane refused to let her diagnosis define her.

Initially, Jane felt isolated, unsure of where to turn. She tried to continue her usual routines, but her increasing fear of falling left her less active and more withdrawn. After a few months, she knew she needed to act, so she reached out to a local osteoporosis support group. This decision changed her life.

Jane started attending weekly exercise classes designed for people with osteoporosis. The instructor introduced her to weight-bearing exercises and Tai Chi, which improved her balance, strength, and confidence. Additionally, Jane found a sense of community in the group. Sharing her fears and triumphs with others who truly understood her experience helped Jane regain control of her life.

Through her journey, Jane also focused on her diet, working with a nutritionist to incorporate more calcium-rich foods and ensure she was getting enough vitamin D. She took small steps—adjusting her daily routine to include healthier meals and finding ways to stay active within her limits.

Key Takeaways:

- Joining a support group and participating in osteoporosis-specific exercise programs can enhance both physical and emotional well-being.
- A strong support network, including professionals like nutritionists, can help develop a tailored health plan that complements medical treatment.
- Small, consistent lifestyle changes, such as adjusting your diet and engaging in safe physical activity, are crucial to managing osteoporosis

Michael - A Firefighter's Path to Recovery and Prevention

Michael, a 64-year-old retired firefighter, was no stranger to physical challenges. However, when a seemingly small slip on wet pavement resulted in a hip fracture, he was diagnosed with osteoporosis. Like many men, Michael had never considered that he might be at risk. The diagnosis felt like a heavy blow to his self-image as a strong, physically capable man.

After surgery to repair his hip, Michael's doctor recommended a bone density scan, which confirmed that he had osteoporosis. Initially frustrated and discouraged, Michael had to confront the fact that this condition would require significant lifestyle adjustments.

Determined to regain his strength, Michael began working with a physical therapist to create a structured exercise routine that included resistance training and balance exercises. He focused on low-impact activities like swimming and cycling, which helped him rebuild muscle without putting too much strain on his bones.

Michael also made important dietary changes. He increased his intake of calcium and magnesium-rich foods, such as leafy greens, nuts, and seeds, and began taking vitamin D supplements as his doctor advised. Additionally, he stopped smoking—a habit he'd struggled with for years—recognizing how it weakened his bones.

Michael's experience as a firefighter had taught him resilience, and he applied that same determination to his osteoporosis journey. Over time, he not only recovered from his fracture but also became a strong advocate for men's bone health, encouraging others to get screened and make bone health a priority.

Key Takeaways:

- Men are often unaware of their risk for osteoporosis, making regular bone density screenings necessary for early diagnosis.
- Recovery from a fracture requires both physical therapy and lifestyle changes, such as improving diet and quitting harmful habits like smoking.
- Strength and resilience come from physical capability and the determination to make long-term changes that support bone health.

Maria - Traditional Wisdom Meets Modern Medicine

At 70, Maria was diagnosed with osteoporosis after experiencing multiple minor fractures. Raised in a family that valued traditional remedies, she was initially hesitant to rely on medications. However, her fractures made it clear that she needed a plan that combined both her cultural heritage and modern treatment options.

Maria sought guidance from her healthcare provider but also consulted with an Ayurvedic practitioner, who introduced her to natural herbs like ashwagandha and turmeric to support her bone health. Maria integrated these into her routine, alongside her prescribed medication, and noticed improvements in her overall well-being.

In addition, Maria embraced yoga to improve her balance and flexibility. Although she had learned yoga in her youth, she had not practiced it regularly for years. As part of her osteoporosis management, she rediscovered the gentle poses that helped strengthen her muscles and joints without putting excessive pressure on her bones.

Her approach blended traditional remedies with medical guidance, proving that you don't have to choose one over the other. With her doctor monitoring her progress, Maria safely integrated her Ayurvedic supplements while adhering to her prescribed treatments.

Key Takeaways:

- Blending traditional remedies with modern medical treatments can offer a holistic approach to managing osteoporosis.
- Consulting with healthcare providers to ensure safety is critical when incorporating natural supplements alongside prescription medication.
- Gentle exercises like yoga can be highly beneficial for maintaining balance, flexibility, and overall bone health, especially for older adults.

Imani - Advocacy Through Adversity

Imani, a vibrant 37-year-old woman, was diagnosed with osteoporosis due to a rare genetic condition. The diagnosis came after a fracture from a fall during a simple jog—a wake-up call for Imani, who had always been physically active. Unlike most people with osteoporosis, Imani's youth made the diagnosis even more unexpected, and she struggled with the stigma of having a condition typically associated with older adults.

Imani initially felt angry and frustrated but quickly turned her emotions into advocacy. She created a blog to share her story and connect with others who, like her, faced the emotional and physical challenges of osteoporosis at a younger age. Her blog gained traction, and soon, she had a supportive online community that shared resources, tips, and stories of resilience.

With her doctor's support, Imani developed a comprehensive treatment plan that included bisphosphonates to strengthen her bones and strength training exercises to enhance her muscle mass. She also focused on maintaining a balanced calcium-rich diet, opting for plant-based sources due to her lactose intolerance.

Imani's advocacy work has empowered many others with osteoporosis to share their stories and actively manage their health. She thrives by balancing her treatment plan with her passion for raising awareness.

Key Takeaways:

- Younger individuals with osteoporosis may face unique emotional challenges, including stigma and isolation, but advocacy and community can provide support.
- Raising awareness and sharing personal experiences can empower others to take control of their health.
- A tailored treatment plan, including medication, exercise, and dietary modifications, can help younger individuals manage osteoporosis effectively.

Ayesha - Bridging Cultures to Find Balance

Ayesha, a 58-year-old woman of Middle Eastern descent, was diagnosed with osteoporosis after her doctor noticed signs of significant bone loss during a routine checkup. Having grown up in a family where traditional health remedies were commonly used, Ayesha felt conflicted about starting medication.

Her doctor recommended bisphosphonates to manage her condition, but Ayesha wanted to explore natural remedies first. She consulted her family, who suggested trying calcium-rich seeds like sesame and chia, staples in her cultural diet. Ayesha incorporated these into her meals and fortified plant-based milk as she struggled with lactose intolerance.

To address her concerns about mobility and balance, Ayesha took inspiration from Middle Eastern dance, also known as belly dancing. She found a local class and discovered that the gentle movements improved her core strength and flexibility, reducing her risk of falls. This cultural connection helped her physically and emotionally, reconnecting her to a part of her identity.

Ayesha's ability to combine modern treatments with cultural practices allowed her to find a balance that worked for her. She continues to thrive today, blending her traditional values with modern osteoporosis care.

Key Takeaways:

- Cultural traditions can offer valuable insights and tools for managing bone health, especially when combined with modern treatments.
- Movement-based activities, like dance, can improve balance and strength while providing emotional and cultural benefits.
- Exploring a mix of traditional and modern remedies can lead to a personalized, effective osteoporosis management plan.

John - Late Diagnosis and the Path to Recovery

At 67, John's active lifestyle was abruptly interrupted by a fall that resulted in a fractured vertebra. It wasn't until this incident that he was diagnosed with osteoporosis, a condition he had unknowingly lived with for years. For John, the late diagnosis felt like a setback, but he was determined to rebuild his health.

John worked closely with his healthcare provider to develop a comprehensive recovery plan. This included taking anabolic medications to stimulate bone growth and enrolling in a physical rehabilitation program to rebuild his strength and mobility. He also began incorporating Tai Chi into his routine to improve his balance and prevent future falls.

As part of his new lifestyle, John adopted a plant-based diet rich in calcium, magnesium, and vitamin D. He swapped out his usual fast-food meals for home-cooked dishes featuring leafy greens, beans, and fortified alternatives.

Over time, John's dedication to his treatment and lifestyle changes helped him recover his mobility and confidence. He now advocates for early osteoporosis screening, particularly for men, to ensure others don't face

Monitoring Bone Health

Regular monitoring is essential for managing osteoporosis, as it provides crucial insights into your bone health over time. The DEXA (Dual-Energy X-ray Absorptiometry) scan, considered the gold standard for measuring bone mineral density (BMD), is recommended every two years for postmenopausal women and men over 70. This simple, non-invasive scan helps assess the current state of your bones, providing valuable information on whether your bone density is improving, stabilizing, or declining. For individuals at higher risk, such as those with a history of fractures, specific medical conditions, or long-term steroid use, more frequent monitoring may be necessary. This allows for early detection of any adverse changes and timely adjustments to the treatment plan.

However, while the DEXA scan is vital, it's only one piece of the puzzle. Bone turnover markers, which are proteins or enzymes found in your blood or urine, offer additional insights into the rate at which your bones are breaking down and rebuilding. These markers help assess whether the treatment effectively slows bone loss or increases bone formation. For instance, C-telopeptide (CTX) and procollagen type 1 N-terminal propeptide (P1NP) are commonly measured markers that indicate the activity of bone turnover. Monitoring these markers provides an earlier indicator of how well your body is responding to therapy, often before changes in bone density are visible on a DEXA scan.

In addition to these tests, regular physical exams are an essential component of managing osteoporosis. Your healthcare provider will assess factors such as posture, mobility, balance, and overall strength. These assessments are particularly important for identifying changes that might increase the risk of falls and fractures. A physical exam can also help detect spinal deformities, such as kyphosis, which can result from vertebral fractures associated with osteoporosis.

Furthermore, your doctor may evaluate other health factors that contribute to bone health, such as hormone levels (particularly in postmenopausal women), calcium and vitamin D levels, and overall nutritional status. These routine assessments allow your healthcare team to take a holistic approach, ensuring that all contributing factors to bone health are addressed, whether through medication, supplements, lifestyle adjustments, or dietary changes.

Regular monitoring not only tracks progress but also empowers you to make informed decisions about your treatment. Whether it's deciding when to intensify therapy, exploring new treatment options, or making small adjustments to your routine, having a clear picture of your bone health enables proactive management of osteoporosis. Regular communication with your healthcare provider is key, as they will interpret these results in the context of your overall health, adjusting your treatment plan as needed to ensure the best outcomes.

By staying vigilant with DEXA scans, bone turnover markers, and physical exams, you're taking a proactive step in protecting your bone health and minimizing the risk of fractures, giving you greater control over your osteoporosis management.

Discussing Results with Your Doctor

When it comes to managing osteoporosis, conversation with your doctor about your test results is crucial. Preparing for your appointment can help you get the most out of this discussion. Start by noting down any specific questions you may have about your recent tests. For instance, understanding the difference between T-scores and Z-scores can be confusing but is essential for assessing your bone health. The T-score compares your bone density to that of a healthy young adult, while the Z-score compares it to people of your age, gender, and size. Knowing what these numbers mean in relation to your overall bone health will help you understand the severity of your condition and guide decisions about your treatment.

It's also important to share any new or worsening symptoms you've experienced, such as back pain or height loss, which can be indicative of vertebral fractures—a common yet sometimes silent consequence of osteoporosis. These symptoms provide important context that your doctor will consider when assessing your overall bone health. Even subtle changes in posture or unexplained pain should be discussed, as they could signal underlying issues that might not appear immediately on a DEXA scan.

Beyond the physical aspects, it's essential to address the emotional impact of living with osteoporosis openly. Many individuals find the diagnosis overwhelming, often feeling anxious about the possibility of fractures or changes in their independence. Let your doctor know if you're feeling anxious, fearful, or even depressed about managing your condition. They may be able to provide resources such as counseling or support groups that can help you manage the emotional toll of osteoporosis. Addressing these concerns also ensures that your treatment plan accounts for your mental and physical well-being.

When reviewing your results, be proactive in discussing the next steps for your treatment. Ask about potential treatment options, whether they involve medication, supplements, or more holistic approaches like physical therapy. Discuss the benefits and possible side effects of any prescribed medications, and don't hesitate to bring up any lifestyle changes you could make to complement your medical treatment. For example, you might ask about incorporating weight-bearing exercises or adjusting your diet to improve calcium and vitamin D intake. Collaborating with your doctor on these lifestyle changes ensures that your treatment plan is well-rounded and tailored to your individual needs.

If you're uncertain about any recommendations, don't be afraid to seek a second opinion. It's vital that you feel confident and comfortable with the course of treatment you're pursuing. A second opinion can provide reassurance or offer new insights that could enhance your care.

Lastly, if you feel that additional therapies—like physical therapy—could benefit your mobility, balance, or overall strength, suggest these options to your doctor. Physical therapy is often an invaluable resource in helping manage osteoporosis, particularly in preventing falls and improving muscle strength, both of which can reduce the risk of fractures. Your doctor can help coordinate these services and ensure they are covered as part of your treatment plan.

By preparing for your appointment, asking the right questions, and advocating for your health, you can have a productive conversation with your doctor and more effectively manage osteoporosis.

Chapter 3: Medical Treatments and Alternatives

I remember when my mom first experienced severe osteoporosis symptoms. It was a difficult time for our family. We spent hours discussing her treatment options, navigating a maze of medical information, and trying to make sense of terms that were new and overwhelming. The fear of what this condition could mean for her future was daunting, but we knew we had to face it head-on.

The process started with a series of appointments. Her doctor explained the various medical treatments available, from bisphosphonates and hormone therapies to newer options like biologics. Each came with its benefits and potential side effects, leaving us with decisions that felt as weighty as the diagnosis itself. For my mom, it wasn't simply a matter of swallowing a pill or taking an injection; she wanted to fully understand what each treatment meant for her overall health, not just her bones.

We quickly learned that managing osteoporosis went beyond the doctor's office. It wasn't just about choosing a medication; it was about understanding the condition in total—how her lifestyle might need to change, the long-term effects, and how she could stay active and independent despite the challenges. Dietary changes became a cornerstone of her plan. We researched foods rich in calcium, magnesium, and vitamin D, creating meals that felt less like a chore and more like an empowering step toward healing.

I hadn't fully anticipated the emotional toll of osteoporosis. I saw how my mom grappled with the fear of falling or the frustration of needing to adjust her daily routines. It wasn't just her bones that needed strengthening—her confidence did, too. We explored alternatives like yoga and tai chi, which not only improved her balance and strength but also became a source of relaxation and mindfulness.

It took time for her to come to terms with the diagnosis. I remember how we sat together, combing through materials on treatment plans and alternatives, wondering if there were natural remedies she could try or lifestyle adjustments that might help lessen the impact of osteoporosis. Herbal remedies like red clover and black cohosh surfaced in our research, though we knew they needed to be approached cautiously. We also found studies on the potential of supplements like collagen and probiotics to support bone health, which became a point of hope in our journey.

This experience reminded me that managing osteoporosis is deeply personal. It's not just about picking the proper medication—it's about addressing the emotional, mental, and physical adjustments that come with such a diagnosis. Every decision felt like a puzzle piece, slowly coming together to create a picture of resilience and adaptability. My mom's journey showed me that the path to managing osteoporosis isn't one-size-fits-all—it's as unique as the individuals it affects.

Overview of Osteoporosis Medications

Osteoporosis treatments fall into several main categories: bisphosphonates, selective estrogen receptor modulators (SERMs), calcitonin, and parathyroid hormone analogs. Each works differently to improve bone mass.

1. **Bisphosphonates** are the most commonly prescribed medications. They slow down bone resorption (bone breakdown), helping maintain or improve bone density. Common bisphosphonates include alendronate (Fosamax), risedronate (Actonel), and ibandronate (Boniva), which are available in tablet form or as injections.
2. **Selective Estrogen Receptor Modulators (SERMs)**, such as Raloxifene (Evista), act like estrogen in bones without affecting other tissues. SERMs reduce bone resorption, particularly useful for postmenopausal women who cannot take hormone replacement therapy (HRT).
3. **Calcitonin** is a hormone that regulates calcium levels and prevents bone resorption. Synthetic calcitonin (like Miacalcin and Fortical) is available as a nasal spray or injection, making it easy to use when other treatments aren't suitable.
4. **Parathyroid hormone analogs**, such as Teriparatide (Forteo) and Abaloparatide (Tymlos), are unique because they stimulate bone formation. These daily injections are especially effective for patients with severe osteoporosis or multiple fractures.

Types of Osteoporosis Medications

Medication Type	Common Brands	Mechanism of Action	Administration
Bisphosphonates	Fosamax, Actonel, Boniva	Slows bone resorption	Oral tablets or injections
SERMs	Evista	Acts like estrogen in bones, reduces bone loss	Oral tablets
Calcitonin	Miacalcin, Fortical	Inhibits bone resorption	Nasal spray or injection
Parathyroid hormone analogs	Forteo, Tymlos	Stimulates new bone formation	Daily injections

Understanding how each medication works will help you and your healthcare provider make informed decisions about managing osteoporosis.

Choosing the right osteoporosis medication depends on factors like overall health, osteoporosis severity, and personal preferences. Options range from daily tablets to monthly injections or nasal sprays, all aimed at improving bone density and preventing fractures, allowing you to stay active.

Osteoporosis medications, such as Fosamax (a bisphosphonate), have been shown to reduce vertebral fractures by 50% and hip fractures by nearly 40%. These medications can significantly improve bone density, especially during the first year of treatment.

However, side effects are a consideration. Common issues include gastrointestinal discomfort, such as nausea or heartburn. Rare but serious risks include atypical femoral fractures (spontaneous thigh bone fractures) and osteonecrosis of the jaw (bone death in the jaw, often related to dental procedures). Regular monitoring through bone density tests (like DEXA scans) and blood tests for calcium levels is essential to track treatment effectiveness and prevent complications.

Extended use of medications, like bisphosphonates, often involves a "drug holiday" after five years to minimize risks, though high-risk patients may need more prolonged treatment. A drug holiday requires careful supervision, with routine check-ups to ensure bone health remains stable.

Anabolic Therapies for Bone Building

Anabolic therapies like Teriparatide (Forteo) and Abaloparatide (Tymlos) are administered through easy-to-use daily injections, usually for up to two years. These treatments stimulate bone formation by activating osteoblasts (cells that form new bone), significantly increasing bone mineral density, especially in the hip and spine. The improvements lead to fewer fractures and a better quality of life. However, there are some long-term safety concerns, such as the rare risk of osteosarcoma (bone cancer), though this hasn't been reported in humans at the recommended dosage.

While anabolic therapies are highly effective, they are expensive, and not all insurance plans fully cover the cost. Since the treatment lasts only two years, patients must switch to antiresorptive drugs afterward to maintain the new bone density gains.

Natural Supplements: Calcium and Vitamin D

Calcium is vital for bone health, as 99% of it is stored in bones. The recommended daily intake for adults is 1,000–1,200 mg. Vitamin D enhances calcium absorption, with a daily recommendation of 600–800 IU for adults. Sources include sunlight, fortified foods, and supplements.

Calcium supplements come in two forms: calcium carbonate, which requires food for absorption, and calcium citrate, which is easier to absorb and can be taken on an empty stomach. Vitamin D3 is more effective than D2 in raising vitamin D levels. When taking supplements, be mindful not to take them with iron-rich foods or medications that may interfere with absorption.

Despite myths, moderate calcium supplementation does not typically cause kidney stones. Drinking enough water and avoiding excess salt helps reduce risks. Always consult your doctor to avoid interactions between supplements and medications.

Balancing Medication with Natural Remedies

Combining medication with natural remedies can effectively manage osteoporosis, enhancing the benefits of both treatments while promoting a holistic approach to bone health. Medications like bisphosphonates are designed to slow bone loss and increase bone density, providing a critical foundation for osteoporosis management. However, their effectiveness can be significantly enhanced when paired with a calcium-rich diet and adequate vitamin D intake. Calcium and vitamin D work synergistically to support bone structure, and they are readily available in dietary sources like leafy greens, dairy products, fortified foods, or supplements when needed. Together, these nutrients help maximize the medication's ability to rebuild and fortify bones.

Similarly, selective estrogen receptor modulators (SERMs) are most effective when combined with regular physical activity. Weight-bearing exercises such as walking, hiking, or resistance training stimulate bone formation while improving balance and muscle strength. Low-impact activities like yoga and Tai Chi also enhance coordination, reduce the risk of falls, and provide added mental health benefits.

An individualized treatment plan is essential to achieving the best results when balancing pharmacotherapy with natural remedies. Regular consultations with healthcare providers ensure that medications, dietary adjustments, and lifestyle changes are tailored to your specific needs. This holistic approach allows both interventions to work harmoniously, optimizing bone health while fostering a sustainable and active lifestyle.

By integrating medication with natural strategies, individuals with osteoporosis can manage the condition effectively and improve overall quality of life. This dual approach emphasizes the importance of treating the body as a whole, supporting long-term health and independence.

Exploring Global Natural Remedies

Traditional practices and natural remedies have been developed around the world to support bone health and complement conventional osteoporosis treatments. These approaches, often rooted in centuries of cultural wisdom, provide unique insights into maintaining strong bones and preventing fractures.

- Traditional Chinese Medicine (TCM): TCM emphasizes holistic balance and often incorporates herbs like ginseng and Rehmannia to strengthen bones and improve overall vitality. Additionally, practices such as Tai Chi combine physical movement with mindfulness to enhance balance, improve muscle strength, and reduce the risk of falls—key benefits for individuals with osteoporosis. Research supports Tai Chi's effectiveness in enhancing stability and preventing fractures, making it a valuable addition to any treatment plan.
- Ayurveda: This ancient Indian practice focuses on harmonizing the body's energies. Herbs such as turmeric, known for its anti-inflammatory properties, and ashwagandha, which supports bone density, are often used in Ayurvedic remedies. Ayurveda also promotes yoga for flexibility, strength, and balance, offering a low-impact way to improve mobility while nurturing the mind-body connection.
- European Herbal Remedies: In Europe, plants like nettles, horsetail, and red clover are traditionally used for their bone-supporting properties. Nettles are rich in calcium and magnesium, while horsetail contains silica, a mineral that helps strengthen the bone matrix. Coupled with the Mediterranean diet—renowned for its emphasis on vegetables, fruits, whole grains, and healthy fats—these remedies offer a nutrient-rich approach to sustaining bone health.

Incorporating these global remedies into your osteoporosis management plan can complement conventional treatments and promote overall well-being. For instance, studies have shown that ginseng may increase bone density, while Tai Chi improves balance and enhances mental clarity, fostering a holistic sense of health.

Before starting any new supplements or practices, always consult your healthcare provider. Quality control is crucial, as not all products meet rigorous safety standards. Begin with low dosages and gradually adjust to suit your needs, ensuring these remedies harmonize with your existing treatments. When approached thoughtfully, global natural remedies can enhance your journey to stronger bones and better health.

Chapter 4: Nutrition for Bone Health

Imagine sitting alone at the dining table, flipping through a photo album. You see your mom, vibrant and full of life, but then remember how osteoporosis later made everyday activities difficult for her. It's in these quiet moments that the connection between diet and bone health becomes undeniable—what we eat directly impacts the strength and resilience of our bones.

Think of bones as living structures that are constantly breaking down and being rebuilt. Like constructing a sturdy house, they need the right materials to remain strong over time. Calcium is the cornerstone, providing the bulk of bone strength, while Vitamin D acts as the foreman, ensuring calcium is absorbed effectively. Beyond these essentials, magnesium and phosphorus play supporting roles, reinforcing the bone matrix. Vitamin K helps to form and maintain bone tissue, while protein serves as the scaffolding that holds everything together. Without these critical nutrients, bones can become brittle, increasing the risk of fractures and making recovery slower and more complicated.

The challenge isn't just knowing what to eat—it's creating a sustainable way to incorporate these nutrients into everyday life. For example, leafy greens like kale, collard greens, and spinach are excellent sources of calcium and magnesium. Fortified plant-based milk or dairy products can fill in any gaps, especially for those who are lactose intolerant or prefer non-dairy options. Fatty fish such as salmon and mackerel provide Vitamin D and omega-3 fatty acids, which support overall bone and joint health. Even tiny seeds like chia and sesame punch above their weight, offering both calcium and magnesium in compact, versatile forms.

Diets like the Mediterranean diet, rich in vegetables, fruits, whole grains, and healthy fats, have emerged as champions for bone health. This way of eating provides a wealth of vitamins and minerals while reducing the intake of bone-depleting substances. In contrast, high sodium levels, often found in processed and fast foods, can leach calcium from the bones, weakening them over time. Caffeine, when consumed in excess, may also contribute to calcium loss, although moderate intake in the context of a well-balanced diet is less concerning.

Hydration, often overlooked, also plays a role in bone health. Staying hydrated supports overall cellular function, including the repair and maintenance of bone tissue. Adding bone-friendly ingredients like a splash of citrus juice to your water can provide Vitamin C, which aids in collagen production—a key component of bone structure.

Reducing processed foods and opting for whole, nutrient-dense options can significantly improve bone strength. Simple substitutions, like replacing refined grains with quinoa or farro, swapping sugary snacks for nuts and dried fruits, or using olive oil instead of butter, can make a tangible difference. Even fermented foods like yogurt and kimchi, rich in probiotics, support gut health, which is increasingly linked to better nutrient absorption and bone density.

Ultimately, the goal isn't just about meeting daily nutrient requirements—it's about creating a dietary pattern that supports your bones throughout your life. Each meal is an opportunity to strengthen your body and prevent the silent progression of osteoporosis. By making informed choices, you can lay the foundation for a future where mobility, strength, and independence remain within your grasp.

Calcium-Rich Foods and How to Include them in your Diet

Dairy products are excellent sources of calcium:

- 1 cup of milk = 300 mg calcium
- 8 oz yogurt = 400 mg calcium
- 1 oz cheddar cheese = 200 mg calcium

Non-dairy options include:

- 1 cup cooked kale = 177 mg calcium
- 1 oz almonds = 75 mg calcium
- 1 tbsp sesame seeds = 88 mg calcium
- 3 oz sardines = 325 mg calcium

Incorporating calcium-rich foods into meals is easy. Add spinach or kale to smoothies, enjoy almond snacks, or use tofu in stir-fries. Here are some recipes for you to try:

Calcium-Rich Smoothie Bowl

This vibrant smoothie bowl is packed with calcium and other essential nutrients for bone health.

Ingredients:

- 1 cup fortified almond milk (450 mg calcium)
- 1/2 cup plain Greek yogurt (100 mg calcium)
- 1/2 cup frozen kale or spinach (30 mg calcium)
- 1/2 banana
- 1/2 cup frozen mixed berries
- 1 tbsp chia seeds (60 mg calcium)
- 1 tbsp almond butter (40 mg calcium)
- 1 tbsp granola (optional for texture)

Instructions:

1. Blend the almond milk, Greek yogurt, kale or spinach, banana, and berries until smooth.
2. Pour into a bowl and top with chia seeds, almond butter, and granola.
3. Serve immediately and enjoy this calcium-rich, energizing start to your day!

Baked Salmon with Sesame Kale

This recipe combines the calcium benefits of leafy greens with the vitamin D from salmon, providing a nutrient-packed meal for bone health.

Ingredients:

- 2 salmon fillets (570 IU vitamin D per serving)
- 4 cups kale, chopped (177 mg calcium per cup)
- 1 tbsp sesame seeds (88 mg calcium)
- 1 tbsp olive oil
- 1 clove garlic, minced
- 1 tbsp lemon juice
- Salt and pepper to taste

Instructions:

1. Preheat the oven to 375°F (190°C). Season the salmon fillets with salt, pepper, and a drizzle of olive oil.
2. Bake the salmon for 15-20 minutes or until it flakes easily with a fork.
3. Meanwhile, sauté the garlic in olive oil over medium heat. Add the chopped kale and cook until wilted, about 3-5 minutes.
4. Sprinkle sesame seeds over the kale and season with lemon juice, salt, and pepper.
5. Serve the baked salmon on a bed of sesame kale.

Chickpea, Spinach, and Quinoa Stir-Fry

This dish is loaded with plant-based calcium and magnesium, ideal for vegans or anyone looking for a nutrient-dense meal.

Ingredients:

- 1 cup cooked quinoa (31 mg calcium)
- 1 can chickpeas, drained and rinsed (210 mg calcium)
- 3 cups spinach, chopped (245 mg calcium)
- 1/2 red bell pepper, sliced
- 1 tbsp olive oil
- 2 garlic cloves, minced
- 1 tsp cumin
- 1/2 tsp paprika
- Salt and pepper to taste

Instructions:

1. Heat the olive oil in a pan over medium heat. Add garlic and sauté until fragrant.
2. Add the bell pepper and cook for 2-3 minutes.
3. Stir in the chickpeas, spinach, cumin, paprika, salt, and pepper. Cook until the spinach is wilted.
4. Mix in the cooked quinoa and stir well to combine.
5. Serve warm, garnished with a sprinkle of fresh herbs, if desired.

Tofu and Broccoli Stir-Fry with Almonds

Tofu, broccoli, and almonds boost calcium in this flavorful and easy-to-make stir-fry.

Ingredients:

- 1/2 block firm tofu, cubed (430 mg calcium)
- 2 cups broccoli florets (86 mg calcium)
- 1/4 cup sliced almonds (75 mg calcium)
- 1 tbsp sesame oil
- 2 tbsp soy sauce (low sodium)
- 1 tsp grated ginger
- 1 garlic clove, minced
- 1 tbsp sesame seeds (optional)
- Cooked brown rice for serving

Instructions:

1. Heat sesame oil in a large pan or wok over medium heat. Add the tofu and cook until golden brown on all sides. Remove and set aside.
2. In the same pan, sauté garlic and ginger for 1 minute.
3. Add the broccoli florets and stir-fry for 5 minutes, until tender but still crisp.
4. Return the tofu to the pan, add soy sauce, and stir to combine.
5. Sprinkle with sliced almonds and sesame seeds (optional) for added crunch and calcium.
6. Serve over brown rice.

Sardine and Avocado Toast

This quick and tasty meal provides a great source of calcium and vitamin D from the sardines and healthy fats from the avocado.

Ingredients:

- 1 can sardines (325 mg calcium)
- 1 ripe avocado
- 2 slices whole grain bread
- 1 tbsp lemon juice
- Salt and pepper to taste
- Red pepper flakes (optional)

Instructions:

1. Toast the bread slices to your liking.
2. Mash the avocado in a bowl, mixing in the lemon juice, salt, and pepper.
3. Spread the avocado mixture on the toast and top with sardines.
4. Sprinkle with red pepper flakes for a spicy kick, if desired.

Almond Butter and Banana Chia Pudding

A calcium-rich dessert that's easy to make and full of bone-boosting nutrients.

Ingredients:

- 1/2 cup chia seeds (300 mg calcium)
- 2 cups almond milk (900 mg calcium)
- 1 tbsp almond butter (40 mg calcium)
- 1 banana, sliced
- 1 tsp vanilla extract
- 1 tsp maple syrup (optional)

Instructions:

1. In a bowl, whisk together chia seeds, almond milk, almond butter, vanilla extract, and maple syrup (if using).
2. Let the mixture sit for 10 minutes, then whisk again to prevent clumping.
3. Cover and refrigerate for at least 4 hours or overnight.
4. Serve topped with banana slices.

These healthy recipes are packed with bone-supporting nutrients like calcium, vitamin D, magnesium, and protein. They're easy to prepare and delicious, making it simple to support bone health through everyday meals.

The Importance of Vitamin D

Vitamin D is essential for absorbing calcium, and its best source is sunlight. Fifteen to twenty minutes of sun exposure a few times a week can provide sufficient vitamin D. Food sources include fatty fish, like salmon, eggs, and fortified foods. However, supplements may be necessary for those living in regions with limited sun exposure.

Sample Meal Plans for Stronger Bones

- **Breakfast**: Fortified cereal with berries and milk (300 mg calcium, 100 IU vitamin D).
- **Lunch**: Salmon salad with greens and almonds (250 mg calcium, 400 IU vitamin D).
- **Dinner**: Kale and almond pesto pasta (350 mg calcium).

Spinach and Feta Stuffed Chicken Breast

This flavorful dish combines lean protein with calcium-rich spinach and feta, making it a perfect dinner for bone health.

Ingredients:

- 2 boneless, skinless chicken breasts
- 1 cup fresh spinach, chopped (60 mg calcium)
- 1/4 cup crumbled feta cheese (100 mg calcium)
- 1 tbsp olive oil
- 1 clove garlic, minced
- Salt and pepper to taste

Instructions:

1. Preheat the oven to 375°F (190°C).
2. Butterfly the chicken breasts by slicing them horizontally without cutting all the way through.
3. Heat olive oil in a pan and sauté garlic until fragrant. Add spinach and cook until wilted.
4. Mix the cooked spinach with feta cheese and stuff the mixture into the chicken breasts. Secure with toothpicks.
5. Place the chicken in a baking dish, season with salt and pepper, and bake for 20-25 minutes or until fully cooked.

Greek Yogurt Parfait with Almonds and Berries

This easy-to-make parfait is rich in calcium, protein, and antioxidants, perfect for breakfast or a snack.

Ingredients:

- 1 cup Greek yogurt (200 mg calcium)
- 1/4 cup granola
- 1/2 cup mixed berries (blueberries, strawberries, raspberries)
- 1 tbsp sliced almonds (75 mg calcium)
- 1 tsp honey (optional)

Instructions:

1. layer Greek yogurt, granola, and berries in a glass or bowl.
2. Top with sliced almonds and drizzle with honey, if desired.
3. Serve immediately for a refreshing and nutritious treat.

Roasted Brussels Sprouts with Tahini Drizzle

This simple side dish packs a calcium punch with the combination of Brussels sprouts and tahini.

Ingredients:

- 2 cups Brussels sprouts, halved (110 mg calcium)
- 1 tbsp olive oil
- Salt and pepper to taste
- 2 tbsp tahini (130 mg calcium)
- 1 tbsp lemon juice
- 1 clove garlic, minced
- 2 tbsp water

Instructions:

1. Preheat the oven to 400°F (200°C). Toss Brussels sprouts with olive oil, salt, and pepper, then spread them on a baking sheet.
2. Roast for 20-25 minutes, until golden and crispy.
3. In a small bowl, whisk together tahini, lemon juice, garlic, and water to make a smooth drizzle.
4. Serve the roasted Brussels sprouts with the tahini drizzle on top.

Calcium-Packed Veggie Pizza

This homemade pizza is a fun and delicious way to sneak in calcium with nutrient-dense toppings.

Ingredients:

- 1 whole-grain pizza crust
- 1/4 cup tomato sauce
- 1/2 cup shredded mozzarella cheese (180 mg calcium)
- 1/2 cup cooked broccoli florets (43 mg calcium)
- 1/4 cup sliced bell peppers
- 2 tbsp grated Parmesan cheese (55 mg calcium)
- 1 tsp Italian seasoning

Instructions:

1. Preheat the oven according to the pizza crust package instructions.
2. Spread tomato sauce evenly over the crust.
3. Sprinkle mozzarella cheese over the sauce, then add broccoli and bell peppers.
4. Top with Parmesan cheese and Italian seasoning.
5. Bake as directed, until the crust is golden and the cheese is bubbly.

Tofu Scramble with Kale and Mushrooms

This vegan-friendly scramble is packed with calcium, magnesium, and protein to support bone health.

Ingredients:

- 1/2 block firm tofu, crumbled (430 mg calcium)
- 2 cups kale, chopped (177 mg calcium)
- 1/2 cup mushrooms, sliced
- 1 tbsp olive oil
- 1/4 tsp turmeric
- 1/4 tsp paprika
- Salt and pepper to taste

Instructions:

1. Heat olive oil in a skillet over medium heat. Add mushrooms and cook until softened.
2. Stir in kale and cook until wilted.
3. Add crumbled tofu, turmeric, paprika, salt, and pepper. Cook for 5-7 minutes, stirring frequently.
4. Serve hot, paired with whole-grain toast or avocado slices, for a hearty, nutrient-packed breakfast or lunch.

Sweet Potato and Black Bean Tacos

These flavorful tacos provide plant-based calcium and vitamin C for better calcium absorption.

Ingredients:

- 1 medium sweet potato, diced (40 mg calcium)
- 1 cup canned black beans, drained and rinsed (50 mg calcium)
- 2 cups chopped spinach (122 mg calcium)
- 1 tbsp olive oil
- 1 tsp cumin
- 1/2 tsp chili powder
- 4 small corn tortillas
- 2 tbsp plain Greek yogurt (50 mg calcium)
- Lime wedges for serving

Instructions:

1. Preheat the oven to 400°F (200°C). Toss diced sweet potato with olive oil, cumin, and chili powder. Roast for 20 minutes or until tender.
2. Heat black beans in a pan over low heat.
3. Warm tortillas and layer with roasted sweet potato, spinach, and black beans.
4. Drizzle with Greek yogurt and serve with lime wedges.

Sardine Pasta with Lemon and Capers

This simple pasta dish offers a boost of calcium and vitamin D from sardines.

Ingredients:

- 1 can sardines, drained (325 mg calcium)
- 8 oz whole-grain spaghetti
- 1 tbsp olive oil
- 2 garlic cloves, minced
- 1 tbsp capers
- 1 tbsp lemon juice
- 1/4 cup Parmesan cheese, grated (110 mg calcium)
- Salt and pepper to taste

Instructions:

1. Cook spaghetti according to package instructions. Drain and set aside.
2. Heat olive oil in a skillet over medium heat. Sauté garlic until fragrant.
3. Add sardines, breaking them into pieces with a fork. Stir in capers and lemon juice.
4. Toss the cooked spaghetti in the skillet and mix well. Top with Parmesan cheese before serving.

Cottage Cheese and Berry Bowl

A quick and refreshing snack loaded with calcium and antioxidants.

Ingredients:

- 1 cup cottage cheese (200 mg calcium)
- 1/2 cup mixed berries (blueberries, strawberries, raspberries)
- 1 tbsp chia seeds (60 mg calcium)
- 1 tsp honey

Instructions:

1. In a bowl, layer cottage cheese and mixed berries.
2. Sprinkle with chia seeds and drizzle with honey.
3. Enjoy as a snack or light breakfast.

Broccoli and Cheddar Soup

This creamy soup is rich in calcium and vitamin K, essential for bone health.

Ingredients:

- 2 cups broccoli florets (86 mg calcium per cup)
- 1/2 cup shredded cheddar cheese (200 mg calcium)
- 2 cups low-sodium vegetable broth
- 1 cup milk (300 mg calcium)
- 1 tbsp olive oil
- 1/2 onion, diced
- 1 clove garlic, minced
- Salt and pepper to taste

Instructions:

1. Heat olive oil in a pot over medium heat. Sauté onion and garlic until softened.
2. Add broccoli and vegetable broth. Simmer until broccoli is tender, about 10 minutes.
3. Blend the soup until smooth using an immersion blender. Stir in milk and cheddar cheese until melted.
4. Season with salt and pepper before serving.

Kale and White Bean Salad

A quick and nutritious salad that combines calcium-rich kale with protein-packed beans.

Ingredients:

- 3 cups kale, chopped (177 mg calcium per cup)
- 1 cup canned white beans, drained and rinsed (100 mg calcium)
- 1/4 cup crumbled feta cheese (100 mg calcium)
- 1 tbsp olive oil
- 1 tbsp lemon juice
- Salt and pepper to taste

Instructions:

1. In a large bowl, massage kale with olive oil and lemon juice until tender.
2. Add white beans and feta cheese. Toss to combine.
3. Season with salt and pepper before serving.

Almond and Fig Overnight Oats

This make-ahead breakfast is a delicious way to start the day with calcium and fiber.

Ingredients:

- 1/2 cup rolled oats
- 1 cup almond milk (450 mg calcium)
- 1 tbsp almond butter (40 mg calcium)
- 2 dried figs, chopped (25 mg calcium)
- 1 tsp vanilla extract

Instructions:

1. In a jar or bowl, combine oats, almond milk, almond butter, figs, and vanilla extract.
2. Stir well, cover, and refrigerate overnight.
3. Serve cold or warm the next morning.

Spinach and Ricotta Stuffed Shells

A satisfying meal rich in calcium and iron from spinach and ricotta.

Ingredients:

- 12 jumbo pasta shells
- 2 cups fresh spinach, chopped (122 mg calcium per cup)
- 1 cup ricotta cheese (240 mg calcium)
- 1/2 cup marinara sauce
- 1/4 cup shredded mozzarella cheese (180 mg calcium)
- 1/4 tsp nutmeg
- Salt and pepper to taste

Instructions:

1. Preheat the oven to 375°F (190°C). Cook pasta shells according to package instructions. Drain and set aside.
2. In a bowl, mix spinach, ricotta cheese, nutmeg, salt, and pepper.
3. Stuff each pasta shell with the spinach-ricotta mixture. Place in a baking dish and top with marinara sauce and mozzarella cheese.
4. Bake for 20-25 minutes until bubbly and golden.

Lentil and Sweet Potato Stew

A hearty, calcium-packed stew full of plant-based nutrients.

Ingredients:

- 1 cup red lentils (40 mg calcium)
- 1 medium sweet potato, diced (40 mg calcium)
- 1 cup canned diced tomatoes
- 2 cups low-sodium vegetable broth
- 2 cups kale, chopped (177 mg calcium per cup)
- 1 tbsp olive oil
- 1 tsp turmeric
- 1 tsp cumin
- 1 clove garlic, minced
- Salt and pepper to taste

Instructions:

1. Heat olive oil in a pot over medium heat. Sauté garlic until fragrant.
2. Add sweet potatoes, turmeric, and cumin. Cook for 2–3 minutes.
3. Stir in lentils, tomatoes, and vegetable broth. Simmer for 20 minutes.
4. Add kale and cook until wilted. Season with salt and pepper before serving.

Cabbage and Carrot Slaw with Tahini Dressing

A refreshing slaw that's rich in calcium and vitamins.

Ingredients:

- 2 cups shredded cabbage (40 mg calcium)
- 1 cup shredded carrots
- 2 tbsp tahini (130 mg calcium)
- 1 tbsp lemon juice
- 1 tbsp olive oil
- 1 tsp honey
- Salt and pepper to taste

Instructions:

1. In a large bowl, combine shredded cabbage and carrots.
2. Whisk tahini, lemon juice, olive oil, honey, salt, and pepper in a small bowl.
3. Pour the dressing over the slaw and toss to combine. Serve as a side dish.

Baked Eggplant Parmesan

This calcium-rich dish uses baked eggplant as a healthy base.

Ingredients:

- 1 medium eggplant, sliced (20 mg calcium per cup)
- 1/2 cup marinara sauce
- 1/2 cup shredded mozzarella (180 mg calcium)
- 1/4 cup grated Parmesan cheese (55 mg calcium)
- 1/4 cup breadcrumbs
- 1 tsp Italian seasoning

Instructions:

1. Preheat oven to 375°F (190°C). Arrange eggplant slices on a baking sheet.
2. Top each slice with marinara sauce, mozzarella, Parmesan, breadcrumbs, and Italian seasoning.
3. Bake for 20–25 minutes until cheese is bubbly.

Sesame-Crusted Tofu Nuggets

A crunchy snack packed with plant-based calcium.

Ingredients:

- 1/2 block firm tofu, cubed (430 mg calcium)
- 1/4 cup sesame seeds (352 mg calcium)
- 2 tbsp soy sauce (low sodium)
- 1 tbsp olive oil
- 1/4 tsp garlic powder

Instructions:

1. Preheat oven to 400°F (200°C). Toss tofu cubes with soy sauce and garlic powder.
2. Coat each cube in sesame seeds. Arrange on a baking sheet and drizzle with olive oil.
3. Bake for 15–20 minutes, turning halfway through, until golden.

Baked Oatmeal with Almonds and Berries

A warm, calcium-rich breakfast that's easy to prepare in advance.

Ingredients:

- 2 cups rolled oats (120 mg calcium)
- 2 cups almond milk (450 mg calcium)
- 1/2 cup sliced almonds (150 mg calcium)
- 1 cup mixed berries
- 1 tsp vanilla extract
- 1 tsp cinnamon

Instructions:

1. Preheat oven to 375°F (190°C). Combine all ingredients in a large mixing bowl.
2. Pour the mixture into a greased baking dish.
3. Bake for 25–30 minutes until set. Serve warm or cold.

Swiss Chard and Mushroom Frittata

A nutrient-dense dish packed with calcium and vitamin D.

Ingredients:

- 4 eggs
- 1/2 cup Swiss chard, chopped (50 mg calcium)
- 1/2 cup sliced mushrooms
- 1/4 cup shredded cheddar (100 mg calcium)
- 1 tbsp olive oil
- Salt and pepper to taste

Instructions:

1. Preheat oven to 350°F (175°C). Heat olive oil in an oven-safe skillet over medium heat.
2. Sauté mushrooms and Swiss chard until softened.
3. Beat eggs, mix with cheddar, and pour into the skillet.
4. Bake for 15 minutes or until the frittata is set.

Orange and Almond Salad

A light and refreshing salad with a calcium boost from almonds.

Ingredients:

- 1 large orange, segmented
- 4 cups mixed greens (40 mg calcium)
- 1/4 cup sliced almonds (75 mg calcium)
- 2 tbsp olive oil
- 1 tbsp balsamic vinegar
- Salt and pepper to taste

Instructions:

1. In a large bowl, combine orange segments, mixed greens, and almonds.
2. Drizzle with olive oil and balsamic vinegar. Toss gently and serve.

Spaghetti Squash with Creamy Tahini Sauce

A low-carb dish packed with calcium and healthy fats.

Ingredients:

- 1 medium spaghetti squash
- 2 tbsp tahini (130 mg calcium)
- 1 tbsp lemon juice
- 1 clove garlic, minced
- 1/4 cup water
- 1/4 tsp paprika
- Salt and pepper to taste

Instructions:

1. Preheat oven to 400°F (200°C). Cut the squash in half and roast for 40 minutes.
2. In a small bowl, whisk tahini, lemon juice, garlic, water, paprika, salt, and pepper.
3. Scrape squash strands with a fork and toss with the tahini sauce.

Creamy Polenta with Roasted Vegetables

A comforting dish full of calcium and flavor.

Ingredients:

- 1 cup polenta (30 mg calcium)
- 2 cups milk (600 mg calcium)
- 1/2 cup Parmesan cheese (110 mg calcium)
- 1 cup roasted vegetables (zucchini, bell peppers, or broccoli)
- 1 tbsp olive oil
- Salt and pepper to taste

Instructions:

1. Heat milk in a saucepan and slowly whisk in polenta. Cook until creamy, about 10 minutes.
2. Stir in Parmesan cheese and season with salt and pepper.
3. Top with roasted vegetables and serve warm.

Indian-Style Spinach and Paneer Curry (Saag Paneer)

A classic Indian dish packed with calcium from spinach and paneer (Indian cottage cheese).

Ingredients:

- 2 cups fresh spinach, chopped (245 mg calcium)
- 1 cup paneer cubes (150 mg calcium)
- 1 medium onion, finely chopped
- 2 garlic cloves, minced
- 1 tsp grated ginger
- 1/2 tsp turmeric
- 1/2 tsp cumin seeds
- 1/2 cup plain Greek yogurt (100 mg calcium)
- 1 tbsp olive oil
- Salt to taste

Instructions:

1. Heat olive oil in a pan and sauté cumin seeds until aromatic. Add onion, garlic, and ginger; cook until golden.
2. Stir in turmeric and spinach. Cook until wilted, then blend into a smooth paste (optional).
3. Add paneer cubes and Greek yogurt, and simmer for 5 minutes. Season with salt before serving with rice or naan.

Mediterranean Chickpea and Tahini Salad

This Middle Eastern-inspired salad combines chickpeas and tahini for a creamy, calcium-rich dish.

Ingredients:

- 1 can chickpeas, drained and rinsed (210 mg calcium)
- 1/4 cup tahini (260 mg calcium)
- 1 tbsp lemon juice
- 1 clove garlic, minced
- 2 cups mixed greens (40 mg calcium)
- 1/2 cup cherry tomatoes, halved
- 1 tbsp olive oil
- Salt and pepper to taste

Instructions:

1. Whisk tahini, lemon juice, garlic, and olive oil in a small bowl to make the dressing.
2. Toss chickpeas, mixed greens, and cherry tomatoes in a large bowl.
3. Drizzle with the tahini dressing and season with salt and pepper before serving.

Japanese Miso Soup with Tofu and Wakame

A simple Japanese soup rich in calcium from tofu and seaweed.

Ingredients:

- 4 cups water
- 2 tbsp miso paste
- 1/2 block firm tofu, cubed (430 mg calcium)
- 1/4 cup dried wakame seaweed (40 mg calcium)
- 2 green onions, sliced

Instructions:

1. Bring water to a boil and stir in miso paste until dissolved.
2. Add tofu and wakame, and simmer for 5 minutes.
3. Garnish with green onions before serving.

Mexican Black Bean and Avocado Tostadas

A crispy and flavorful Mexican dish with plant-based calcium.

Ingredients:

- 4 small corn tortillas
- 1 cup black beans, mashed (50 mg calcium)
- 1 avocado, sliced
- 1/4 cup shredded cheddar cheese (100 mg calcium)
- 1/2 cup shredded lettuce
- 1 tbsp lime juice
- 1 tsp chili powder

Instructions:

1. Toast corn tortillas until crispy.
2. Spread mashed black beans over each tortilla and top with avocado slices.
3. Sprinkle with cheddar cheese, lettuce, lime juice, and chili powder.

Greek Spanakopita (Spinach Pie)

This Greek pastry combines flaky phyllo dough with a calcium-rich spinach and feta filling.

Ingredients:

- 2 cups fresh spinach, chopped (245 mg calcium)
- 1/2 cup crumbled feta cheese (200 mg calcium)
- 1/4 cup ricotta cheese (120 mg calcium)
- 1 clove garlic, minced
- 6 sheets phyllo dough
- 2 tbsp olive oil

Instructions:

1. Preheat oven to 375°F (190°C).
2. Sauté garlic and spinach until wilted. Let cool, then mix with feta and ricotta cheese.
3. Brush phyllo sheets with olive oil and layer them in a baking dish. Add the spinach mixture and fold the phyllo over to seal.
4. Bake for 25–30 minutes until golden and crispy.

West African Peanut Stew

A rich and creamy stew with calcium from peanuts and leafy greens.

Ingredients:

- 1 cup peanut butter (176 mg calcium)
- 2 cups chopped kale (177 mg calcium per cup)
- 1 sweet potato, diced (40 mg calcium)
- 1 can diced tomatoes
- 2 cups vegetable broth
- 1 clove garlic, minced
- 1 tsp paprika
- 1 tbsp olive oil
- Salt and pepper to taste

Instructions:

1. Heat olive oil in a pot and sauté the garlic. Add sweet potatoes and paprika and cook for 5 minutes.
2. Stir in tomatoes, peanut butter, and vegetable broth. Simmer until sweet potatoes are tender.
3. Add kale and cook until wilted. Season with salt and pepper before serving.

Italian White Bean and Kale Bruschetta

A flavorful Italian appetizer combining calcium-rich beans and kale.

Ingredients:

- 1 can white beans, drained and rinsed (100 mg calcium)
- 2 cups kale, chopped (177 mg calcium)
- 1 clove garlic, minced
- 1 tbsp olive oil
- 4 slices whole-grain bread
- 1 tbsp balsamic vinegar

Instructions:

1. Heat olive oil in a pan and sauté garlic. Add kale and cook until wilted.
2. Stir in white beans and balsamic vinegar. Cook for 2–3 minutes.
3. Toast bread slices and top with the bean and kale mixture. Serve warm.

Korean Kimchi Fried Rice

This Korean dish combines tangy kimchi with calcium-rich sesame seeds and greens.

Ingredients:

- 2 cups cooked brown rice
- 1/2 cup kimchi, chopped
- 1/2 cup spinach, chopped (60 mg calcium)
- 1 tbsp sesame oil
- 1 tbsp soy sauce (low sodium)
- 1 tbsp sesame seeds (88 mg calcium)
- 1 egg (optional, for topping)

Instructions:

1. Heat sesame oil in a skillet over medium heat. Add kimchi and cook for 2 minutes.
2. Stir in rice, spinach, and soy sauce. Cook until heated through.
3. Sprinkle with sesame seeds and top with a fried egg, if desired.

Ensure meals include a balance of protein, carbohydrates, and healthy fats, along with essential nutrients for bone health.

Supplements can help when dietary intake is insufficient, especially for those with dietary restrictions. Choose high-quality supplements that provide clear information about dosage and ingredients. It's recommended that adults get 1,000–1,200 mg of calcium and 600–800 IU of vitamin D daily. Always consult your healthcare provider before starting new supplements to avoid potential interactions with medications.

Research shows that calcium and vitamin D supplementation effectively reduce fracture risk, especially in older adults. However, experts emphasize that nutrients from food are generally more beneficial than supplements, as they contain additional nutrients that work synergistically to improve health.

Chapter 5: Exercise and Mobility

Imagine standing at the edge of a beautiful forest, excited to explore the winding trails ahead, but a small voice inside you whispers, "What if you fall?" This fear of fractures can turn even the simplest activities into daunting challenges when living with osteoporosis. It's natural to feel hesitant, but the good news is that exercise is one of the most powerful tools available to help strengthen your bones, boost your overall health, and regain the confidence to live a full and active life.

Gaining confidence through exercise doesn't happen overnight, but with a well-structured, consistent routine, you'll begin to notice improvements in both your physical strength and your mental resilience. Each small victory—whether it's walking a little farther or standing a little taller—helps break the cycle of fear, allowing you to engage with the world around you without constant anxiety about fractures or falls.

The Importance of Physical Activity

Exercise is critical for maintaining bone health, acting like a natural medicine for your bones. Weight-bearing and resistance exercises stimulate bone growth by putting stress on your bones, prompting them to grow denser and stronger. This process, known as stress-induced bone growth, is essential for preserving bone density and slowing the progression of osteoporosis. As you lift weights, your muscles become stronger to handle the load. Similarly, when you engage in weight-bearing exercises, your bones adapt to stress, reducing the risk of fractures.

Beyond bone health, regular physical activity offers numerous other benefits. Improved cardiovascular health lowers the risk of heart disease, and stronger muscles support and protect bones in daily activities. Exercises that improve balance and coordination, like yoga and Tai Chi, are particularly valuable because they reduce the risk of falls, a major concern for osteoporosis patients.

Getting started with exercise can be intimidating, especially if you're worried about injury. The key is to begin gently and build your strength over time. Low-impact exercises such as walking, swimming, or cycling are excellent starting points because they improve cardiovascular fitness while being easy on the joints and bones. Incorporating flexibility exercises like stretching or yoga into your routine will also help you avoid stiffness and maintain a full range of motion, which is essential for mobility.

To stay motivated, set realistic goals. For instance, start walking for 20 minutes three times a week and gradually increase the duration and frequency as you build endurance. An exercise partner can also keep you accountable and make the experience more enjoyable. Logging your workouts in a journal or app allows you to track your progress and see how far you've come, which can be encouraging when motivation dips.

Remember, consistency is key. Exercise for bone health is a long-term commitment, not a quick fix. Find activities you enjoy, whether it's dancing, yoga, or gardening, and stick with them. The more you move, the more your bones will benefit.

Weight-Bearing Exercises Explained

Weight-bearing exercises are the foundation of maintaining bone strength. These activities require your bones to support your body weight and work against gravity, which encourages your bones to become stronger and denser. There are two types of weight-bearing exercises: high-impact and low-impact.

High-impact exercises include activities like running, jumping, or dancing. These exercises are highly effective for building bone density but may not be suitable for everyone, especially those with advanced osteoporosis or joint issues. For many, low-impact exercises such as walking, hiking, or using an elliptical machine provide similar benefits without the risk of injury.

One of the simplest and most effective weight-bearing exercises is walking. Walking at a brisk pace promotes bone health without requiring special equipment or a gym membership. You can walk outdoors on a treadmill or even indoors at home. Hiking offers an additional challenge by incorporating varied terrains, which engage different muscles and stimulate bone growth in the lower body. Dancing is another enjoyable weight-bearing activity that combines fun with fitness—whether you prefer ballroom, salsa, or freestyle dancing in your living room, you're building bone density while improving coordination.

As with any exercise, proper technique is essential. Ensure you maintain good posture while walking or hiking: keep your shoulders back, head up, and arms swinging naturally. Wear supportive shoes to absorb impact and protect your joints. Starting with a five-minute warm-up and ending with a cool-down stretch will help prevent injury and ease muscle tension.

For those who need extra support or have mobility concerns, walking poles can offer stability and distribute body weight more evenly, reducing strain on your bones and joints. If you prefer exercising indoors, an elliptical machine provides a low-impact, joint-friendly alternative that still challenges your bones. You can adjust the resistance and incline as you build strength, making this a versatile tool for weight-bearing exercise.

Balance and Coordination Training

Balance and coordination are crucial, especially for those with osteoporosis, as they help prevent falls, which can lead to fractures. Strong stabilizing muscles and improved proprioception—the body's ability to sense its position in space—are key to maintaining balance and preventing injuries. Incorporating targeted balance exercises into your routine can enhance your stability and confidence in daily activities.

Begin with simple exercises like standing on one leg. This may sound easy, but it engages your stabilizing muscles, improving balance over time. Stand near a sturdy surface, like a chair or countertop, for support. Shift your weight onto one leg and lift the other leg slightly off the ground. Hold this position for 10 seconds or longer, depending on your ability. As you progress, try balancing without assistance and aim to increase your hold time gradually. To make the exercise more challenging, incorporate dynamic movements like lifting and lowering the raised leg or extending it forward or backward.

Another excellent balance exercise is the heel-to-toe walk. Imagine walking in a straight line, placing the heel of one foot directly in front of the toes of the other foot. This exercise mimics walking on a balance beam and strengthens both balance and coordination. Focus on controlled, slow movements to ensure proper technique. To increase difficulty, try walking backward or closing your eyes briefly (only if it's safe to do so).

Consider Tai Chi, which combines slow, flowing movements with focused breathing for a more holistic approach. Tai Chi is particularly beneficial for balance, coordination, and mental focus, making it ideal for individuals with osteoporosis. Its low-impact nature reduces the risk of strain or injury and can be adapted to suit any fitness level. Regular practice has been shown to enhance proprioception, improve posture, and increase lower-body strength. Tai Chi sessions often include movements like the "single whip" and "brush knee," which gently challenge balance and flexibility.

If Tai Chi doesn't resonate, other options like yoga or Pilates offer similar benefits. Yoga poses like the tree pose or Warrior III emphasize balance, while Pilates strengthens the core, a crucial stability component. These practices build physical strength and improve mindfulness, helping you feel more grounded and in control.

Balance training can also be incorporated into daily activities. For example, brushing your teeth while standing on one leg or walking slowly while carrying a light object can engage your stabilizing muscles. Even small adjustments to your routine, like taking stairs instead of elevators, help enhance coordination and balance over time.

By dedicating 10–15 minutes daily to balance and coordination exercises, you can significantly reduce your risk of falls, improve your overall stability, and enhance your quality of life. Small, consistent efforts lead to meaningful progress, empowering you to navigate daily activities confidently.

Safe and Effective Strength Training

Strength training is another critical component of osteoporosis management. By building muscle strength, you create a support system for your bones, reducing their load during everyday movements. This not only helps prevent fractures but also enhances mobility and independence.

There are many ways to engage in strength training safely. Resistance bands are versatile tools that allow you to adjust the intensity of your workout. Exercises like bicep curls, leg lifts, and shoulder presses can easily be performed with resistance bands at home. Bodyweight exercises like squats and push-ups are also effective and can be done anywhere. Start with modified versions if needed, and gradually increase intensity as you build strength.

When using weights, begin with light dumbbells and focus on proper form. For example, keep your feet shoulder-width apart, back straight, and knees aligned with your toes when doing squats. To protect your joints, avoid letting your knees move past your toes. Push-ups, whether performed on your knees or a wall, help strengthen your upper body without overloading your bones.

The key to safe strength training is gradual progression. Start with lower resistance or lighter weights and increase as you become stronger. Always listen to your body and take breaks if you experience pain or discomfort.

Yoga and Pilates offer a unique blend of strength, flexibility, and balance training, making them ideal for people with osteoporosis. These practices improve core strength, supporting the spine and enhancing stability, while increasing joint flexibility and range of motion.

In Yoga, the Tree Pose improves balance and strengthens the legs. In this pose, you stand on one leg, with the other foot resting on your inner thigh or calf. It's a simple yet effective way to build strength while enhancing focus and concentration. Pilates, on the other hand, focuses on core stability and controlled movements. Exercises like the Bridge Pose strengthen the glutes, hamstrings, and lower back, all of which are important for supporting the spine and pelvis.

Both Yoga and Pilates incorporate mindfulness and controlled breathing, helping reduce stress—a key factor in managing osteoporosis. Stress increases cortisol levels, which can negatively impact bone health, so these practices offer both physical and mental benefits.

The Warrior pose builds leg strength and enhances balance. Move one foot back, bend the front knee and stretch your arms overhead. The Bridge pose supports the back and glutes while stretching the chest and spine. Rest on your back with your knees bent and feet flat on the floor, and raise your hips towards the roof. In Pilates, pelvic tilts support the lower back and abdominal muscles. Lie on your back with your knees bent and feet resting on the floor, and slowly tilt your pelvis upward. Leg circles boost hip mobility and strengthen the core. Lie on your back with one leg raised towards the roof and make small, controlled circles. The modified plank supports the core and upper body. Start on your hands and knees, then extend one leg at a time to form a straight line from your head to your heels, maintaining the position while engaging your core.

Safety Adaptations in Yoga and Pilates

When practicing yoga or Pilates, safety is key to preventing injury and ensuring you're reaping the benefits without putting undue stress on your bones. Yoga props, such as blocks, straps, and bolsters, can be incredibly helpful for those with osteoporosis, as they allow you to maintain proper alignment and modify poses to suit your ability level.

For example, in the Tree Pose, where you stand on one leg to improve balance, you can place a yoga block under your hand for additional support. This stabilizes you as you improve your balance without the risk of falling. Straps can also be beneficial in poses like Seated Forward Bend, where they help you reach your feet without straining your back. These simple tools ensure you get the most out of your yoga practice while staying safe.

However, it's essential to avoid certain poses that can put too much stress on your spine, particularly deep twists, forward bends, or any exercise that involves rounding the back. These movements can compress the vertebrae and increase the risk of fractures. Instead, focus on gentle, controlled movements that build strength and stability, such as seated poses or standing postures with modifications.

Luckily, many resources are available to help you safely begin yoga and Pilates, even if you're new to exercise. Look for programs designed specifically for osteoporosis that provide clear instructions and modifications for various poses. Online platforms can offer Yoga and Pilates, beginner-friendly classes designed with osteoporosis in mind. By choosing the right resources and making adjustments, yoga and Pilates can become an integral part of your exercise routine, helping to improve flexibility, strength, and balance while protecting your bones.

Creating a Personalized Exercise Plan

A personalized exercise plan tailored to your fitness level and goals can be transformative in managing osteoporosis. The first step in developing your plan is assessing your fitness level. Consider any physical limitations, past injuries, or health concerns that might impact your ability to exercise. For example, if you've recently recovered from a fracture or surgery, your plan should start with low-impact activities to avoid putting stress on weakened bones. Consulting a healthcare provider or physical therapist can also provide valuable insight into what exercises are safe and beneficial for your condition.

Once you clearly understand your starting point, it's time to set realistic, achievable goals. Setting specific, measurable goals will keep you focused and motivated. Instead of simply saying, "I want to exercise more," try a goal like, "I will walk for 20 minutes, three times a week," or, "I will complete 10 minutes of balance exercises every morning." Goals like these are clear, trackable, and flexible, allowing you to celebrate progress and make adjustments as needed.

Incorporating different types of exercises into your plan is also essential. A well-rounded plan includes weight-bearing exercises for bone health, such as walking, dancing, or stair climbing. Balance exercises, like standing on one leg or practicing Tai Chi, are crucial for reducing the risk of falls, while strength training with resistance bands or light weights builds muscle to support your bones. Flexibility exercises, like yoga or gentle stretching, enhance mobility and help maintain a full range of motion. Variety not only ensures that you're working on all areas of fitness but also keeps your routine engaging and prevents overuse injuries that can result from repeatedly doing the same type of exercise.

To stay consistent, schedule your workouts as part of your daily routine. Consider joining a class or finding an exercise buddy to make the experience more enjoyable and hold yourself accountable. With a personalized plan that suits your needs and preferences, managing osteoporosis becomes a proactive and empowering part of your lifestyle.

Your Personal Movement Journey

Navigating exercise with osteoporosis isn't about pushing limits—it's about understanding your body and moving smartly. This chapter is your roadmap to creating a sustainable, safe, and effective exercise routine that supports your bone health and overall well-being.

Myth-Busting: Exercise and Osteoporosis

Common misconceptions can prevent people from achieving optimal health. Let's address some prevalent myths:

- **Myth**: Exercise is too risky with osteoporosis
- **Reality**: Targeted, appropriate exercise is one of the most powerful tools for managing bone health
- **Myth**: You're too old to start exercising
- **Reality**: It's never too late to improve strength, balance, and bone density

Practical Exercise Planning: A Step-by-Step Guide

Step 1: Professional Consultation

Before beginning any exercise program:

- Schedule a comprehensive medical assessment
- Discuss your specific bone density measurements
- Get personalized recommendations from:
    - Your primary care physician
    - Endocrinologist
    - Physical therapist specializing in bone health
    - Certified osteoporosis fitness trainer

What to Discuss in Your Consultation

- Current bone density status
- Fracture history
- Medication interactions
- Existing mobility limitations
- Personal fitness goals

Step 2: Assessing Your Current Fitness Level

Self-Assessment Checklist

1. Can you stand on one leg for 10 seconds?
2. Do you experience pain during light activities?

3. How many stairs can you climb without resting?
4. Can you sit and stand from a chair without using your hands?

Pro Tip: Don't get discouraged by current limitations. These are starting points, not finish lines.

Step 3: Creating Your Personalized Exercise Toolkit

Equipment Recommendations

Budget-Friendly Options:

- Resistance bands ($10-$20)
- Yoga mat ($15-$30)
- Light dumbbells (2-5 lbs)
- Stability ball
- Comfortable, supportive shoes

Home Exercise Space

- Clear, open area
- Non-slip flooring
- Nearby chair for support
- Good lighting
- Water bottle
- Optional: Full-length mirror

Step 4: Building Your Weekly Exercise Routine

Beginner's Weekly Template

Monday: Balance and Flexibility

- 15-minute gentle yoga
- 10-minute balance exercises
- Stretching

Tuesday: Strength Training

- Resistance band exercises
- Light dumbbell work
- Chair-supported movements

Wednesday: Rest and Recovery

- Gentle walking
- Light stretching
- Deep breathing exercises

Thursday: Cardiovascular Health

- 30-minute walking
- Low-impact dancing
- Swimming (if available)

Friday: Strength and Balance

- Repeated Tuesday's routine
- Add new variations

Saturday: Enjoyable Movement

- Gardening
- Gentle hiking
- Social dance class

Sunday: Active Recovery

- Stretching
- Meditation
- Light walking

Progression Strategies

Beginner Level (0-3 Months)

- Focus on form and consistency
- Use support (chairs, walls)
- Start with 10-15 minute sessions

- Prioritize safety over intensity

Intermediate Level (3-6 Months)

- Increase session duration
- Add light weights
- Introduce more complex movements
- Improve balance challenges

Advanced Level (6-12 Months)

- Implement progressive resistance
- Try group fitness classes
- Explore more dynamic exercises
- Work with specialized trainer

Safety Red Flags: When to Stop

Immediately cease exercise and consult your healthcare provider if you experience:

- Sharp, stabbing pain
- Sudden weakness
- Dizziness
- Chest discomfort
- Unusual fatigue
- Breathing difficulties

Technology and Exercise Support

Recommended Apps

- Silver Sneakers
- Fitbit Senior Fitness
- AARP Fitness App
- Yoga for Seniors
- Balance Training Platforms

Tracking Progress

- Take monthly measurements
- Photograph exercise forms
- Keep a mobility journal
- Note energy levels and mood changes

Psychological Aspects of Exercise

Motivation Techniques

- Set small, achievable goals
- Celebrate every milestone
- Join support groups
- Share your journey with family
- Be kind to yourself

Mental Health Benefits

- Reduced anxiety
- Improved self-confidence
- Enhanced social connections
- Sense of empowerment
- Stress reduction

Your Movement, Your Power

Exercise with osteoporosis isn't about perfection—it's about progression. Each movement celebrates what your body can do, not a punishment for what it can't.

Remember: You're not just exercising to prevent bone loss. You're building strength, confidence, and a vibrant life.

Recommended Resources

- Local osteoporosis support groups
- Senior fitness centers
- Online exercise communities
- Certified osteoporosis fitness trainers

Staying Motivated and Consistent

Sticking to an exercise plan can be difficult, but there are ways to stay motivated. Keeping an exercise journal is a great strategy for tracking progress and reflecting on your achievements. Write down your workouts, how you felt before and after, and any improvements you notice. This record can be a powerful motivator when you look back and see how far you've come.

Celebrating small milestones is another excellent way to stay engaged with your routine. Whether it's walking an extra five minutes or lifting a heavier weight, these achievements are worth celebrating. Reward yourself with something enjoyable, like new workout gear or a relaxing activity, to keep your motivation high.

Joining an exercise group or class can also be incredibly helpful. Exercising with others who share similar goals provides accountability and support. Look for community or online classes designed for individuals with osteoporosis. These classes often include modifications for all fitness levels and are led by instructors who understand the unique needs of people with bone health concerns.

As we wrap up this chapter, remember that a personalized and consistent exercise routine is one of the most powerful tools for managing osteoporosis. Combining weight-bearing exercises, balance training, and strength workouts can support your bones, improve mobility, and protect yourself from fractures. With safety adaptations like yoga props and personalized modifications, you can exercise confidently, knowing you're minimizing risks.

Exercise is not just about physical health; it also boosts mental well-being and enhances quality of life. As you embark on this journey, remember that consistency, patience, and enjoyment are the keys to success. With a well-rounded approach and a commitment to staying active, you'll be well on your way to stronger bones and a more vibrant, active life.

In the next chapter, we'll explore how to create a safe home environment that further reduces the risk of falls and injuries, ensuring that you continue to live independently and confidently.

Chapter 6: Preventing Falls and Injuries

Imagine relaxing in your cozy living room, enjoying a cup of tea, when you notice your favorite rug bunched at the edge. It's a small thing, easy to overlook, but in that moment, you realize it could be dangerous. You've heard stories of people tripping and falling, and with osteoporosis, the risk is even higher. A simple stumble could lead to a serious fracture. Suddenly, what was once a comfortable home begins to feel like a source of anxiety. But it doesn't have to be this way. By making a few thoughtful adjustments, you can transform your home into a safe space that reduces the risk of falls, ensuring you feel secure in every room.

Home Safety Modifications

Common household hazards are often hidden in plain sight, presenting risks we might not immediately notice. Loose rugs and carpets, for example, can easily slip or bunch up, turning into tripping hazards. Picture yourself walking through the living room; your foot catches on the corner of a rug, and suddenly, you're on the floor. Another risky area is cluttered walkways. Shoes, magazines, and electrical cords left in the path can create unnecessary dangers. Then there's the bathroom—wet, slippery floors from showers or sinks are particularly hazardous for falls.

To address these risks, start by securing loose rugs with non-slip pads. These pads grip the floor, keeping rugs in place and reducing the chance of them shifting. For carpets, ensure they're firmly attached to the floor. Consider replacing high-pile rugs with low-pile options that are less likely to catch your feet, reducing the risk further.

Clearing clutter from walkways is another simple but essential step. Designate a space for shoes near the entrance, use cable organizers to manage electrical cords, and ensure that items like magazines have a proper place. Consider creating designated "no-clutter zones" in high-traffic areas, such as hallways, doorways, and near staircases, where tripping risks are higher.

Proper lighting is another key factor in preventing falls. Hallways, staircases, and frequently used rooms should be well-lit, with bright, energy-efficient bulbs providing consistent illumination. Motion-sensor night lights are an excellent addition, as they turn on automatically when movement is detected, guiding you safely through your home at night. Smart lighting systems can allow you to control brightness and timing with voice commands or a smartphone app, ensuring you never walk into a dark room. Use light switches that are easily accessible and glow in the dark for added convenience.

Fall-Proofing Your Living Space

Each room in your home presents unique challenges, but with a few strategic changes, you can dramatically reduce your fall risk. Let's take a closer look at key rooms in the home:

- **Kitchen**: Keep frequently used items within easy reach to avoid unnecessary stretching or climbing. Store heavy or bulky objects at waist height to reduce strain. Use non-slip mats near the sink and stove for added stability. Avoid standing on chairs or unstable stools to reach high shelves—use a sturdy step stool with a handrail instead. Consider rearranging items periodically to ensure your kitchen remains accessible as your needs evolve.
- **Bedroom**: Position your nightstand close to the bed for easy access to essentials like glasses, medication, and phones. Use a lamp with a touch sensor or an easy-to-reach switch for nighttime visibility. Ensure the area around your bed is free from loose mats or cords that could trip you. Bed risers can make getting in and out of bed easier, and adjustable beds may provide additional comfort and safety. Motion-activated lights under the bed can softly illuminate the floor, guiding your steps during nighttime trips.
- **Living Room**: Arrange furniture to create clear, open walkways, avoiding low tables or footstools that could obstruct your path. If you have a coffee table, make sure it's sturdy with rounded corners to prevent injuries if you bump into it. Secure any loose cords from electronic devices using cable organizers. Replace unstable or wobbly furniture with more secure options.

Assistive Devices and Technology

For those with osteoporosis, assistive devices can be crucial in enhancing safety and independence. Common devices like canes and walkers provide essential stability, allowing you to confidently move around. Grab bars and handrails in key locations, such as the bathroom and stairways, offer extra support when standing up or navigating tricky spaces. Reachers and grabbers are another useful tool, allowing you to pick up objects without needing to bend over.

Technology has also provided us with new ways to stay safe. Fall detection devices can automatically sense a fall and alert emergency contacts, while smart home systems let you control lights, thermostats, and alarms using voice commands or mobile apps. These technologies can provide added peace of mind and convenience.

When choosing assistive devices, consult with your healthcare provider to ensure you select the right tools for your specific needs. Proper fitting is essential for canes and walkers—your elbow should be slightly bent when you hold the handle. Grab bars must be securely installed into wall studs for maximum stability.

Regular maintenance of assistive devices is crucial. For canes and walkers, check for wear on rubber tips and replace them as needed. For smart devices, keep the software updated to ensure proper functioning.

Safe Movement and Daily Activities

Everyday movements like getting in and out of bed or standing up from a chair require extra attention when you have osteoporosis. To get out of bed safely, start by sitting on the edge with your feet flat on the floor, then use your hands to push yourself into a standing position. When sitting down or standing up from a chair, use the armrests for support, and always move slowly to maintain your balance.

Stairs are another common area of concern. Always use handrails for support, and take your time, placing your whole foot on each step before moving to the next. Shoes with non-slip soles are essential for indoor and outdoor activities, providing extra traction and reducing the risk of slipping.

Emergency Preparedness for Falls

While we take every precaution to prevent falls, it's essential to be prepared in case they do happen. Keep emergency contacts easily accessible in several locations around your home. Having a phone within reach at all times is crucial, whether it's a cell phone, cordless phone, or medical alert system.

Learning how to get up safely after a fall is also important. If you can, roll onto your side, then use your hands and knees to crawl to a sturdy piece of furniture, such as a chair, to help yourself stand. If you cannot get up, use your phone or medical alert device to call for help.

Importance of Routine Vision and Hearing Checks

Good vision and hearing play a critical role in fall prevention. Poor eyesight can make it difficult to detect obstacles, and hearing impairments might prevent you from noticing hazards like a family member calling out a warning or the sound of an approaching object. Regular check-ups with an optometrist and audiologist can ensure your senses are sharp, reducing the likelihood of accidents. Update your prescription glasses if needed, and consider wearing hearing aids if recommended.

Practicing Mindful Movement

Mindfulness isn't just for relaxation—it can help prevent falls, too. Moving with intention makes you more likely to notice potential hazards and maintain your balance. For example:

- Always look ahead while walking instead of focusing on the ground.
- Pause before transitioning positions, such as standing up from a chair or bed.
- Avoid rushing, particularly on stairs or uneven surfaces.

In the next chapter, we will discuss the importance of emotional support and well-being.

Chapter 7: Emotional Well-being and Support

Imagine yourself sitting in your doctor's office, heart racing as you await your latest bone density test results. The doctor enters, sits down, and speaks the words you've dreaded: "You have osteoporosis." Suddenly, a wave of emotions hits—shock, denial, and fear of the future. This chapter delves into handling these emotions and discovering how to thrive emotionally while living with osteoporosis.

The initial emotional response to an osteoporosis diagnosis can be overwhelming. Feelings of shock, denial, or fear about the future are normal. It's difficult to accept that your bones aren't as strong as they once were, especially if you've led an active life. Thoughts like, *This can't be happening to me* or doubts about the diagnosis may flood your mind. Taking time to process the news is essential.

Concerns about future health, fractures, or lifestyle changes can create anxiety. Activities you once enjoyed may now seem risky, and you may wonder how to adjust. While these worries can feel overwhelming, know that many people continue to live fulfilling lives with osteoporosis.

Journaling can be an excellent way to process these emotions. Writing your thoughts down provides clarity, helping you manage worries. Talking to a trusted friend or family member can also offer emotional support. Simply knowing someone is listening can make a significant difference.

If you need deeper emotional guidance, seeking professional counseling may help. A therapist can help you work through complicated feelings and build resilience. A healthcare provider or local resources can help you find a counselor who specializes in chronic illness.

Be kind to yourself during this time. Avoid self-blame, as osteoporosis is influenced by many factors outside your control. Self-care practices—whether a warm bath, reading, or spending time outdoors—can be small yet meaningful acts of self-kindness. Mindfulness and breathing exercises also help ease anxiety, grounding you in the present.

Hobbies and activities you love can also offer a sense of normalcy. Whether playing an instrument, gardening, or painting, these moments of joy remind you that osteoporosis doesn't define your life.

Reflection Section: Self-Compassion Practice

Take a moment to reflect on the activities that bring you joy and peace. List three self-care activities that you genuinely enjoy—whether it's reading a book, taking a warm bath, or going for a walk in nature—and commit to incorporating them into your weekly routine. These activities may seem simple, but they are essential in maintaining your emotional well-being and helping you manage the challenges of osteoporosis.

Remember, self-care isn't indulgent; it's an act of kindness toward yourself, a way to recharge and restore balance in your life. These small but meaningful moments help reduce stress, foster a positive mindset, and remind you that caring for yourself is just as important as any medical treatment. By consistently carving out time for self-care, you nurture your mental and emotional resilience, which in turn supports your physical health and overall quality of life.

Consider setting reminders or scheduling these moments into your week—just as you would with any important appointment. Taking this time for yourself is not a luxury; it is vital in sustaining your energy, focus, and well-being as you navigate your osteoporosis journey.

Building a Support Network

An osteoporosis diagnosis can initially feel isolating, but building a strong support network can lighten the load. Social support is crucial for emotional well-being. When surrounded by people who understand your journey, the burden of managing osteoporosis feels lighter.

Begin with family and friends. Often, loved ones want to help but aren't sure how. Have an honest conversation about your needs—whether it's attending doctor visits, running errands, or simply offering a listening ear. Don't hesitate to ask for specific support.

Community groups, either local or virtual, provide an excellent opportunity to connect with others who understand what you're going through. Look for osteoporosis support groups or chronic illness groups through hospitals or community centers. These spaces offer shared experiences, valuable advice, and emotional support.

In today's digital age, online communities are a valuable resource. Online platforms, forums, and support apps offer a chance to connect with people worldwide, providing comfort and encouragement. These spaces can be helpful if you prefer sharing anonymously or need advice on managing symptoms, treatment options, or emotional challenges.

Healthcare professionals also play a vital role in your support network. Regular check-ins with your doctor can help you stay on top of your treatment plan. At the same time, mental health professionals can offer tools to manage anxiety or depression related to osteoporosis. A physical therapist can help with mobility, and a nutritionist can guide your dietary needs.

Assertive communication is key to maintaining a strong support network. Be clear about how you're feeling and what type of support you need. Specific requests, such as asking for help with grocery shopping or needing to talk, make it easier for others to provide meaningful help. And remember to express gratitude—small gestures of appreciation go a long way in nurturing relationships.

Interactive Element: Support Network Checklist

Take a few moments to create a list of people you can rely on for support in your life. Think about family members, close friends, healthcare professionals, and community resources that can offer help during your osteoporosis journey. These individuals can provide emotional comfort, practical assistance, or expert guidance as you manage your condition. Remember, you don't have to face osteoporosis alone—your support network is there to lift you up when needed.

Consider expanding your network by reaching out to someone new, whether it's a healthcare provider you haven't consulted yet, a local support group, or even a trusted neighbor. Growing your circle of support can provide fresh perspectives, new ideas, and different types of assistance you may not have considered before. A broader network gives you access to more resources, advice, and encouragement, which are crucial in maintaining your physical and emotional well-being.

As you create this list, reflect on each person's value to your life. Whether they provide a listening ear, medical expertise, or companionship, their role is essential in helping you navigate osteoporosis confidently. Keep this list handy, and don't hesitate to lean on your support system—asking for help when needed is a sign of strength, not weakness.

The Role of Mental Health in Physical Health

Mental and physical health are closely linked, especially when managing a condition like osteoporosis. Stress triggers the release of cortisol, a hormone that, when elevated, can weaken bones by increasing bone resorption and slowing bone formation. Prolonged stress can accelerate bone loss, worsening osteoporosis. Conversely, a positive mental state can enhance your body's ability to heal and maintain health. Feeling mentally strong makes you more likely to engage in beneficial activities like exercising, eating well, and staying social.

Effectively managing stress is essential. Begin by identifying your stress triggers, which may include daily frustrations or larger worries, such as financial concerns or health anxieties. Once you pinpoint what's causing stress, you can create strategies to manage it. Simple relaxation techniques, such as deep breathing or progressive muscle relaxation, can be powerful tools for calming the mind and body.

Living with osteoporosis can also bring specific mental health challenges like anxiety or depression, often fueled by the fear of fractures or loss of independence. Recognizing these emotional difficulties early on is key to managing them. Resources like mental health hotlines, counseling services, and online therapy platforms offer support when needed. Apps like Headspace and Calm can also guide you through mindfulness exercises to help reduce stress and improve emotional well-being.

Resource List: Mental Health Resources

- National Alliance on Mental Illness (NAMI) Helpline
- Headspace (Mindfulness and meditation app)
- BetterHelp (Online counseling platform)

Planning for Long-Term Health

Managing osteoporosis is a long-term commitment. Setting realistic health goals—whether maintaining bone density or enhancing mobility—provides direction. Regular checkups, bone density tests, and a flexible approach to treatment and lifestyle will keep you on track.

Make dietary and exercise changes as part of a sustainable lifestyle, ensuring you get enough calcium and vitamin D, remain physically active, and avoid smoking or excessive drinking habits. Use resources such as support groups, healthcare professionals, and online forums to stay Dietary and exercise changes are part of a sustainable lifestyle.

Resource List: Ongoing Support

- Bone Health and Osteoporosis Foundation
- Mayo Clinic
- Local osteoporosis support groups

Celebrating Progress and Setting Future Goals

Recognizing your progress is vital. Whether it's sticking to an exercise routine or seeing an improvement in bone density, acknowledging these milestones helps sustain motivation. Reward yourself with simple joys, like a special outing, sharing progress with loved ones, or reflecting in your journal.

Set new goals to keep pushing forward—whether it's trying a new exercise, joining a support group, or improving your diet. Stay adaptable and celebrate even the smallest victories, as they contribute to your overall success in managing osteoporosis.

Interactive Element: Milestone Celebration Ideas

- Plan a special outing
- Share progress with friends or family
- Reflect on personal growth in a journal

Chapter 8: Staying Informed and Engaged

Picture yourself in your favorite chair, skimming through a magazine, when an article about a breakthrough osteoporosis treatment catches your eye. Your heart races. Could this be the solution you've been seeking? Staying up to date with the latest research and advancements isn't just interesting—it's essential for managing osteoporosis. In a rapidly evolving medical landscape, staying informed can significantly improve your quality of life.

Keeping up with osteoporosis research is more than just being aware of treatment options—it's about empowering yourself to make decisions that align with your evolving health needs. The landscape of osteoporosis management is constantly changing, with new therapies and technological innovations introduced regularly. As patients become more proactive in their care, having a finger on the pulse of research can help you be part of the conversation with your healthcare team, ensuring that your treatment plan is the best available.

Advancements in the field of biotechnology and genetic research are opening new doors for osteoporosis treatment. Researchers are now exploring the role of genetic predisposition to osteoporosis, which may one day lead to personalized treatments based on your DNA. Imagine having access to therapies tailored specifically to your genetic makeup, potentially increasing effectiveness and reducing side effects. Keeping an eye on these developments through trustworthy medical sources can provide you with exciting insights into the future of bone health.

In addition, regenerative medicine is an emerging area of interest in osteoporosis treatment. Stem cell research explores the potential to regenerate damaged bone tissue, offering hope for those with severe osteoporosis. While still in the early stages, clinical trials are underway, and future breakthroughs in this area could drastically change the treatment landscape. Awareness of these pioneering developments might allow you to explore participation in relevant clinical trials or adopt newer therapies as they become available.

Technology is also revolutionizing the way osteoporosis is diagnosed and monitored. Artificial intelligence (AI) in analyzing bone density scans improves the precision of osteoporosis diagnosis. AI algorithms can detect minute changes in bone structure that may be missed by the human eye, leading to earlier interventions and personalized treatment plans. Staying updated with these technological advancements can empower you to ask your healthcare provider about the possibility of incorporating such innovative tools into your care.

Interactive Element: Research Spotlight

- **Biotechnology and Genetics:** Stay informed about genetic predisposition research.
- **Stem Cell Therapies:** Learn about regenerative medicine and clinical trials.
- **AI in Diagnostics:** Explore how artificial intelligence is transforming osteoporosis diagnosis.

Advocacy and Raising Awareness

Beyond staying informed for personal benefit, advocating for osteoporosis awareness can bring about meaningful change. Advocacy doesn't just happen at the government or policy level—it can happen in your community, workplace, or social circles. You have the power to raise awareness, reduce stigma, and promote education about osteoporosis.

Many individuals feel isolated after a diagnosis, but by sharing your story and experiences, you can help others understand that osteoporosis is manageable. Speaking at local health events or writing articles for community newsletters can spread awareness about early detection, lifestyle changes, and available resources. For example, many people don't know that osteoporosis can affect individuals as young as their 30s due to genetic factors or other underlying conditions. Your voice can help highlight that osteoporosis is not just an "older person's disease."

You could also consider advocating for policy changes. Numerous global and national organizations, such as the Bone Health and Osteoporosis Foundation (BHOF) and the International Osteoporosis Foundation (IOF), promote better healthcare policies for osteoporosis screening and treatment. By joining these efforts, you can influence healthcare coverage to ensure more individuals have access to diagnostic screenings and treatments at an affordable rate. Advocacy can include signing petitions, writing to government representatives, or participating in osteoporosis awareness campaigns like World Osteoporosis Day.

Additionally, advocating for improved osteoporosis education in schools, workplaces, and communities can have long-lasting effects. Many people are unaware of the preventive steps they can take early in life, such as engaging in weight-bearing exercises and consuming adequate calcium and vitamin D. By pushing for more comprehensive osteoporosis education, particularly for younger audiences, you can help future generations take control of their bone health early on.

Exploring Cutting-Edge Treatments

The future of osteoporosis treatment holds exciting potential, and it's important to remain open to these innovations. For instance, biophosphonate alternatives are being explored as potential breakthroughs. Current treatments like biophosphonates can slow bone loss, but newer medications may offer more targeted action with fewer long-term side effects. The development of anabolic therapies, which promote bone formation rather than merely slowing its loss, represents a promising area of research.

Monoclonal antibodies are another emerging treatment for osteoporosis. These lab-made molecules can mimic the body's natural defenses and are being used to slow bone resorption while enhancing bone formation. Drugs like romosozumab, a monoclonal antibody, are at the forefront of these advancements. While newer, these treatments are gaining momentum as clinical trials demonstrate their effectiveness in reducing fracture risk.

In addition, hormone replacement therapies (HRT) are evolving, with new formulations being designed to reduce side effects and improve effectiveness. Post-menopausal women, for example, may benefit from these innovations, which can provide a safer alternative to traditional HRT options.

Staying aware of such cutting-edge treatments means you'll be prepared to discuss them with your doctor when they become widely available. Being proactive about incorporating new options into your treatment plan ensures you get the most advanced care possible.

Expanding Lifestyle Modifications Beyond Diet and Exercise

While diet and exercise are cornerstones of osteoporosis management, other, often overlooked lifestyle changes can support bone health. For example, improving your sleep hygiene can have a profound effect on bone metabolism. Studies show that poor sleep can interfere with your body's ability to repair itself, including bone regeneration. Aiming for 7-9 hours of quality sleep, practicing good sleep habits, and addressing issues like sleep apnea can contribute to better bone health.

Reducing stress is another important factor in osteoporosis management. Chronic stress leads to elevated cortisol levels, a hormone that can decrease bone density over time. Mindfulness practices, such as meditation, yoga, or tai chi, improve balance and flexibility and reduce stress, offering dual benefits for both your mind and bones.

Hydration is often underappreciated in the conversation about bone health. Staying hydrated helps your body maintain the right balance of minerals needed for bone density. Ensuring adequate water intake throughout the day supports overall health and enhances the effectiveness of other osteoporosis treatments.

Finally, managing comorbid conditions, such as diabetes or thyroid disorders, is critical. These conditions can affect bone health in complex ways. For instance, uncontrolled diabetes can contribute to bone fragility, and certain thyroid disorders can accelerate bone loss. By keeping these conditions in check through medication, lifestyle adjustments, and regular monitoring, you can help protect your bones.

The Role of Digital Health Tools

Incorporating digital health tools into your osteoporosis management routine is becoming increasingly common. Wearable devices like smartwatches and fitness trackers can track your daily activity, including steps, workouts, and sleep quality, providing valuable insights into your health. Some advanced devices even monitor your heart rate and stress levels, which can help you manage the impact of stress on your bones.

Virtual consultations and telemedicine have also transformed healthcare access. Now, you can consult with osteoporosis specialists from the comfort of your home, making staying engaged with your treatment plan easier without the hassle of in-person appointments. Many healthcare providers are embracing telemedicine as a convenient way to monitor your condition, adjust medications, and answer questions in real-time.

Interactive Element: Digital Tools and Telemedicine

- **Fitness Trackers:** Use wearable devices to monitor your physical activity and sleep quality.
- **Telemedicine:** Schedule virtual appointments with your healthcare team to stay connected.
- **Health Apps:** Explore apps for nutrition tracking, exercise planning, and medication management.

In the next chapter, we'll explore other medical conditions that can co-exist alongside osteoporosis.

Chapter 9: Osteoporosis and Coexisting Conditions

Living with osteoporosis often involves more than simply managing bone health. Many individuals with osteoporosis find themselves facing other health challenges, as certain diseases and conditions can increase the risk of developing osteoporosis or make its management more complex. Understanding these connections can help you and your healthcare provider create a comprehensive plan that supports your entire health picture, whether it's joint issues, digestive concerns, or chronic illnesses. In this chapter, we'll explore some of the most common conditions frequently accompanying osteoporosis, their impact on bone health, and practical strategies for managing them together.

Osteoarthritis (OA) and Osteoporosis: Managing Joint and Bone Health Together

Osteoarthritis (OA) is a common degenerative joint disorder that causes cartilage between bones to break down, leading to joint pain, stiffness, and limited mobility. While OA and osteoporosis are separate conditions, they often coexist, particularly in older adults, complicating physical activity. The pain from OA can make movement challenging, yet inactivity may worsen joint stiffness and accelerate bone density loss in people with osteoporosis.

To manage both conditions together, a tailored approach using low-impact, joint-friendly exercises can effectively promote joint and bone health without undue stress. Water-based activities, like swimming and water aerobics, provide resistance to build muscle and support joint stability while minimizing joint impact. Incorporating gentle strength training with resistance bands helps strengthen the muscles around joints, which reduces OA-related pain, improves stability, and helps prevent osteoporosis-related fractures. Anti-inflammatory foods, including turmeric, berries, and green tea, can further support OA pain management by reducing inflammation and enhancing bone health.

Working with a physical therapist experienced in joint and bone health can be invaluable. They can guide adaptive exercise routines and joint-sparing techniques—such as ergonomic grips or braces—that reduce joint strain and allow for safe, consistent activity. Complementary therapies like acupuncture and therapeutic massage can relieve pain without increasing bone fragility, making them effective for ongoing OA and osteoporosis management.

Rheumatoid Arthritis (RA) and Osteoporosis: Navigating Immune and Bone Health

Rheumatoid arthritis (RA) is an autoimmune disorder that causes joint inflammation, resulting in pain, swelling, and joint deformity over time. Individuals with RA face a higher risk of developing osteoporosis due to both inflammation-related bone loss and the use of corticosteroid medications, which can weaken bones.

Managing RA and osteoporosis together requires a careful balance of anti-inflammatory and bone-supportive practices. Low-impact exercises like cycling, swimming, and gentle stretching (such as yoga) can enhance mobility, reduce joint stiffness, and support bone strength without exacerbating inflammation. Anti-inflammatory diets rich in omega-3 fatty acids, found in fish and flaxseeds, and antioxidants from colorful vegetables can help reduce RA symptoms while promoting bone density.

A rheumatologist can work with a primary care physician to develop a medication plan that balances inflammation control with bone health preservation. Regularly monitoring bone density, especially when taking corticosteroids, is essential. Supplementing with calcium and vitamin D, alongside RA medications, supports bone health. Additionally, complementary therapies like acupuncture and low-impact Pilates can improve joint function, reduce pain, and provide a holistic approach to managing both RA and osteoporosis.

Type 2 Diabetes and Osteoporosis: Balancing Blood Sugar and Bone Health

Type 2 diabetes can increase the risk of osteoporosis due to factors such as higher blood sugar levels and diabetes medications that may impact bone health. Elevated blood sugar can damage bone tissue over time, while some diabetes medications may reduce calcium absorption, leading to increased bone fragility.

To manage both conditions, maintaining stable blood sugar levels while prioritizing bone health is crucial. A diet low in refined sugars and rich in whole grains, leafy greens, and lean proteins can provide sustained energy and support bone density. Weight-bearing exercises like walking and strength training improve insulin sensitivity, stabilize blood sugar, and promote bone growth.

Working closely with an endocrinologist can ensure that diabetes medications are optimized to reduce bone health risks. Regularly monitoring blood sugar levels and bone density enables more personalized treatment adjustments. Weight management, which is essential for blood sugar control, also benefits bone density. Combining diabetes management with osteoporosis-friendly practices, such as low-impact strength training and dietary supplementation, creates a balanced approach that effectively addresses both conditions.

Celiac Disease and Osteoporosis: Supporting Bone Health Through Diet

Celiac disease, an autoimmune disorder triggered by gluten, can significantly impact bone health due to nutrient malabsorption, especially of calcium and vitamin D. This malabsorption leads to a higher risk of osteoporosis, as the body struggles to absorb essential bone-supporting nutrients.

A strict gluten-free diet is fundamental for individuals with both celiac disease and osteoporosis. Nutrient-rich gluten-free grains, like quinoa and brown rice, along with leafy greens and fortified gluten-free products, can provide essential vitamins and minerals. Calcium and vitamin D supplementation may be necessary to ensure bone health, as individuals with celiac disease often have low levels of these nutrients due to absorption issues.

Regular consultations with a dietitian specializing in celiac disease can help monitor nutrient levels and ensure a balanced gluten-free diet that meets bone health requirements. Weight-bearing and strength exercises, such as yoga and resistance band workouts, can further support bone density without causing gastrointestinal distress. Regular monitoring of bone density is also essential to assess the effectiveness of dietary and lifestyle interventions.

Chronic Kidney Disease (CKD) and Osteoporosis: Balancing Bone Health and Kidney Function

Chronic kidney disease (CKD) often coexists with osteoporosis, as impaired kidney function affects the body's ability to process and retain vital minerals, like calcium and phosphorus, crucial for bone health. CKD can also interfere with vitamin D production, decreasing bone density and an elevated fracture risk.

Managing osteoporosis alongside CKD requires close medical supervision to balance bone health with kidney function. A renal-friendly diet—low in phosphorus and sodium and adjusted for protein—can protect the kidneys while supporting bone health. Calcium supplementation should be approached cautiously, as excess calcium can burden the kidneys. Instead, foods that naturally support bone health, like leafy greens, bell peppers, and berries, are recommended.

It is crucial to work with a nephrologist to tailor a bone health plan that considers CKD limitations. Weight-bearing and low-impact exercises like walking and Tai Chi can support bone density without stressing the kidneys. Monitoring calcium, vitamin D, and phosphorus levels regularly helps tailor a balanced approach to managing CKD and osteoporosis.

Depression and Osteoporosis: Prioritizing Mental and Bone Health

Depression is linked to an increased risk of osteoporosis due to hormonal imbalances, lifestyle factors, and some antidepressants that may impact bone density. Individuals with depression often experience lower physical activity and may have difficulty adhering to bone-healthy diets, leading to bone loss over time.

Addressing both conditions requires a comprehensive approach that includes mental and physical health support. Regular exercise, such as walking, yoga, or swimming, has shown benefits for both bone health and mood improvement. Omega-3-rich foods, like salmon and walnuts, along with leafy greens and vitamin D, simultaneously support brain and bone health.

Counseling, cognitive behavioral therapy, and support groups can be invaluable for managing depression. Consulting with a psychiatrist familiar with bone health considerations can help adjust medications as needed. Small lifestyle adjustments, like a consistent sleep schedule and daily outdoor time, can improve mood and support vitamin D production, promoting a balanced approach to managing both depression and osteoporosis.

"No act of kindness, no matter how small, is ever wasted."

– Aesop

Dear Reader,

Thank you for reading **Thrive with Osteoporosis: Your Guide to Prevent Fractures, Build Strength, Improve Balance, Embrace Natural Remedies, and Practice Safe Exercises for Lifelong Mobility**.

This book was written to empower you with knowledge, practical tools, and a variety of healthy recipes to support bone health and overall well-being. I hope it has given you confidence and clarity on your journey toward thriving with osteoporosis.

Your feedback can help others in ways you might not even realize. By sharing your experience, you could:

- **Inspire someone feeling overwhelmed** to take their first steps toward managing osteoporosis.
- **Guide someone searching for natural remedies, safe exercises, and bone-friendly meals.**
- **Create a ripple effect of hope** that reaches countless people navigating similar challenges.

Leaving a review is a simple act of kindness that could transform someone else's life without expecting anything in return.

How to Leave Your Review: It's quick and easy to share your thoughts on **Amazon**:

1. Click on the Link below or scan the QR code.
2. Scroll down to the **Customer Reviews** section on the Amazon page.
3. Click **"Write a customer review"** and share your honest thoughts—what you loved, what was helpful, or how this book made a difference for you.

You don't need to write a long review. Even a few sentences about the recipes, exercises, or tips you found useful can make a significant impact.Thank you for being a part of this mission to empower others to thrive with osteoporosis. Your kindness and generosity mean the world to me.

Warm regards,
Isabella

https://www.amazon.com/review/create-review/?ie=UTF8&channel=glance-detail&asin=B0DS1D952W

Conclusion

As we reach the end of our journey together, let's revisit the key points we've covered in this book. We've explored osteoporosis from multiple angles: understanding how it affects the body, looking at medical treatments, exploring natural remedies, and delving into practical ways to support and enhance bone health through diet, exercise, and emotional resilience. Along the way, we've also touched on the complex interplay between osteoporosis and other health conditions, recognizing how managing one area of health can directly benefit another.

One of the most important takeaways is that osteoporosis can be managed with the right knowledge and tools. Throughout this book, we've emphasized the value of staying informed, working closely with healthcare providers, and taking proactive measures. Knowing your bone density, identifying risk factors, and creating a tailored plan of action can make a powerful difference in how you live with osteoporosis.

Nutrition plays a fundamental role in maintaining bone health, and we've gone into detail about what to eat for optimal bone strength. A diet rich in calcium, vitamin D, and other essential nutrients forms the backbone of bone health. The recipes and meal plans provided offer ways to integrate these nutrients into your everyday routine, making healthy eating both enjoyable and effective. Remember, the choices you make in the kitchen can have a lasting impact on your bone strength and overall vitality.

Exercise has been another cornerstone of our discussion. Weight-bearing and muscle-strengthening activities are critical in supporting bone density and improving mobility. The exercises we've discussed range from simple weight-bearing moves to gentle balance practices, providing something for everyone, regardless of age or fitness level. Building a sustainable exercise routine that gradually increases in intensity can bolster your bones and keep you active.

The emotional and mental aspects of managing osteoporosis are equally important. We explored coping mechanisms, from building a strong support network to using mindfulness techniques that help manage stress. Emotional well-being, after all, is closely tied to physical health, and nurturing a positive outlook can make each step of this journey smoother and more fulfilling.

As you move forward, here's how to keep building on the foundation we've set in this book:

1. **Keep Learning and Stay Involved**
   Medical advancements continue to shape the landscape of osteoporosis care, and staying updated can empower you to make informed decisions. Whether it's a new diagnostic tool, a dietary recommendation, or a treatment option, staying engaged with credible sources and consulting with your healthcare provider ensures that you're always aware of the latest, most effective solutions.
2. **Take Action and Embrace Change**
   Small, consistent changes in diet, exercise, or routine can have a lasting positive impact. From making your home safer to incorporating bone-strengthening foods and exercises into your day, each step is a positive investment in your health. Explore the tips, tools, and resources shared in this book to craft a lifestyle that strengthens your bones and overall well-being.
3. **Stay Committed and Set New Goals**
   Managing osteoporosis is a lifelong commitment, but with dedication, it's entirely possible to lead a fulfilling, active life. Set milestones, celebrate each achievement, and adjust your goals as you progress. Persistence is key to maintaining bone health, building resilience, and enjoying a sense of accomplishment along the way.

This book aims to provide you with a thorough, compassionate guide to managing osteoporosis effectively. My mom's experience navigating this condition taught me a lot about resilience, the importance of being well-informed, and the power of small, deliberate actions. I share her story and what I've learned from it to support you in finding confidence and optimism in your own journey.

Thank you for allowing me to be part of your journey toward stronger bones and a vibrant, healthy life. Remember, you are never alone—there's a supportive community ready to help and encourage you. Stay positive, keep moving forward, and continue confidently embracing each step. You have the strength to meet osteoporosis's challenges head-on and create a life full of vitality and joy.

References

- *Global, regional prevalence, and risk factors ...*
  https://pubmed.ncbi.nlm.nih.gov/35687123/
- *Osteoporosis - Symptoms and causes - Mayo Clinic*
  https://www.mayoclinic.org/diseases-
  conditions/osteoporosis/symptoms-causes/syc-20351968
- *Osteopenia vs. osteoporosis: What is the difference?*
  https://www.medicalnewstoday.com/articles/osteopenia-vs-
  osteoporosis
- *Psychological state, quality of life, and body composition in ...*
  https://www.ncbi.nlm.nih.gov/pmc/articles/PMC2836755/
- *Osteoporosis - Symptoms and causes*
  https://www.mayoclinic.org/diseases-
  conditions/osteoporosis/symptoms-causes/syc-20351968
- *Bone density scan (DEXA scan) - How it is performed - NHS*
  https://www.nhs.uk/conditions/dexa-scan/what-happens/
- *T-Score Vs. Z-Score for Osteoporosis: What the Results Mean*
  https://www.healthline.com/health/t-score-vs-z-score-osteoporosis
- *Osteoporosis: An Update on Screening, Diagnosis ...*
  https://www.ncbi.nlm.nih.gov/pmc/articles/PMC10084730/
- *FDA approves new treatment for osteoporosis in postmenopausal
  women at high risk ...* https://www.fda.gov/news-events/press-
  announcements/fda-approves-new-treatment-osteoporosis-
  postmenopausal-women-high-risk-fracture
- *Adverse Effects of Bisphosphonates: Implications for ...*
  https://www.ncbi.nlm.nih.gov/pmc/articles/PMC2704135/
- *Role of Traditional Chinese Medicine in Bone ...*
  https://www.ncbi.nlm.nih.gov/pmc/articles/PMC9194098/
- *Calcium and vitamin D supplementation in osteoporosis*
  https://www.uptodate.com/contents/calcium-and-vitamin-d-
  supplementation-in-osteoporosis
- *New Insights into Nutrients for Bone Health and Disease*
  https://www.ncbi.nlm.nih.gov/pmc/articles/PMC10303436/

- *Top 15 Calcium-Rich Foods (Many Are Nondairy)*
  https://www.healthline.com/nutrition/15-calcium-rich-foods
- *Vitamin D for Good Bone Health - OrthoInfo - AAOS*
  https://orthoinfo.aaos.org/en/staying-healthy/vitamin-d-for-good-bone-health/
- *The Mediterranean Diet in Osteoporosis Prevention*
  https://www.ncbi.nlm.nih.gov/pmc/articles/PMC7915719/
- *Exercising with osteoporosis: Stay active the safe way*
  https://www.mayoclinic.org/diseases-conditions/osteoporosis/in-depth/osteoporosis/art-20044989
- *Exercising with osteoporosis: Stay active the safe way*
  https://www.mayoclinic.org/diseases-conditions/osteoporosis/in-depth/osteoporosis/art-20044989
- *Pilates for Osteoporosis: Safety, Benefits, and Risks*
  https://www.healthline.com/health/fitness/pilates-for-osteoporosis
- *Exercise for Your Bone Health | NIAMS*
  https://www.niams.nih.gov/health-topics/exercise-your-bone-health
- *What Are the Must-Have Home Modifications for Aging in Place*
  https://www.assistedliving.org/home-modifications-for-seniors-aging-in-place/
- *The Role of Assistive Devices in Preventing Falls at Home*
  https://www.vha.ca/blog/the-role-of-assistive-devices-in-preventing-falls-at-home/
- *Fear of Falling in Older Adults: A Scoping Review ...*
  https://www.ncbi.nlm.nih.gov/pmc/articles/PMC8629501/
- *Living with Osteoporosis: 8 Exercises to Strengthen Your ...*
  https://www.healthline.com/health/managing-osteoporosis/exercises-to-strengthen-your-bones
- *Emotional wellbeing and osteoporosis*
  https://theros.org.uk/information-and-support/osteoporosis/living-with-osteoporosis/everyday-life/emotional-wellbeing-and-osteoporosis/

- *Building a Strong Support System for Chronic Illness ...*
  https://www.lotusmedicalcentre.com.au/building-a-strong-support-system-for-chronic-illness-management/
- *Mental Health: How It Affects Your Physical Health*
  https://www.webmd.com/mental-health/how-does-mental-health-affect-physical-health
- *Living with Osteoporosis and Helping Others - Bone Talk*
  https://www.bonetalk.org/articles/one-mans-journey-living-with-osteoporosis-and-helping-others
- *Five latest advancements in osteoporosis research*
  https://www.labiotech.eu/best-biotech/osteoporosis-research/
- *Bone Health & Osteoporosis Foundation: Home*
  https://www.bonehealthandosteoporosis.org/
- *Efficacy of Osteoporosis Prevention Smartphone App on ...*
  https://www.ncbi.nlm.nih.gov/pmc/articles/PMC7105101/
- *About Clinical Trials*
  https://www.bonehealthandosteoporosis.org/patients/clinical-trials/about-clinical-trials/

www.ingramcontent.com/pod-product-compliance
Lightning Source LLC
Chambersburg PA
CBHW071236020426

42333CB00015B/1492